MW01615072

Osteoporosis

Second Edition

Kenneth G. Saag, MD, MSc
Jane Knight Lowe Professor of Medicine
Division of Clinical Immunology and Rheumatology
University of Alabama at Birmingham

Sarah L. Morgan, MD, MS, RD, CCD
Professor of Medicine
Medical Director, Osteoporosis Prevention
and Treatment Clinic and DXA Facility
University of Alabama at Birmingham

Gregory A. Clines, MD, PhD
Assistant Professor of Medicine and Cell,
Development, and Integrative Biology
Division of Endocrinology, Diabetes, and Metabolism
University of Alabama at Birmingham
Birmingham VA Medical Center

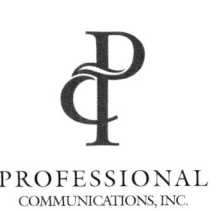

PROFESSIONAL
COMMUNICATIONS, INC.

Copyright 2017
Kenneth G. Saag, MD, MSc,
Sarah L. Morgan, MD, MS, RD,
Gregory A. Clines, MD, PhD

Professional Communications, Inc.

A Medical Publishing & Communications Company

400 Center Bay Drive
West Islip, NY 11795
(t) 631/661-2852
(f) 631/661-2167

PO Box 1427
Durant, OK 74702-1427
(t) 580/745-9838
(f) 580/745-9837

For orders only, please call
1-800-337-9838

or visit our Web site at
www.pcibooks.com

ISBN: 978-1-943236-13-8

Printed in the United States of America

DISCLAIMER

The opinions expressed in this publication reflect those of the authors. However, the authors make no warranty regarding the contents of the publication. The protocols described herein are general and may not apply to a specific patient. Any product mentioned in this publication should be taken in accordance with the prescribing information provided by the manufacturer.

DEDICATION

We dedicate this book to our many colleagues in the bone world and to our patients who have taught us so much and who have inspired us to try and succinctly summarize the current state of this emerging art.

We also dedicate this book to all our families.

ACKNOWLEDGMENT

We wish to thank Professor Juliet Compston for her very helpful edits and input. We also want to thank Sebastian Sattui, MD and Ms. Bridget Alday for their scientific and technical assistance with the book's preparation. We gratefully acknowledge the editors Malcolm Beasley and Phyllis Jones Freeny for their dedicated assistance in seeing this new edition through to completion.

TABLE OF CONTENTS

Introduction: The Society Burden of Osteoporosis — 1

The Physiology of Bone — 2

Pathogenesis of Osteoporosis and
Other Metabolic Bone Diseases — 3

Diagnosis: History, Risk Factors, and
Physical Examination — 4

Diagnosis: Fracture Types, Measuring
Bone Mass, Tests for Secondary Causes, and
Other Methods of Skeletal Assessment — 5

Diagnosis: Biochemical Markers of
Bone Remodeling — 6

Prevention and Treatment:
Nonpharmacologic Therapy — 7

Prevention and Treatment:
Calcium and Vitamin D — 8

Prevention and Treatment:
Pharmacologic Agents — 9

Evolving Pathways and Therapeutic Targets — 10

Osteoporosis in Special Populations — 11

Abbreviations/Acronyms — 12

Index — 13

TABLES

Table 4.1 Conditions, Diseases, and Medications
That Cause or Contribute to Osteoporosis
and Fractures 60

Table 4.2 Risk Factors for FRAX 70

Table 4.3 Physical Examination Findings of
Metabolic and Genetic Bone Disorders 74

Table 5.1 WHO Definitions of Osteoporosis 82

Table 5.2 Laboratory Evaluation of Secondary
Causes of Decreased Bone Mass.............................87

Table 5.3 DXA Best Practice 105

Table 5.4 Indications for Bone Mass Measurement
From the International Society for
Clinical Densitometry 107

Table 5.5 Indications for BMD Coverage From the
US Centers for Medicare and Medicaid
Services (CMS) 109

Table 5.6 Indications for Vertebral Imaging 118

Table 6.1 Biochemical Bone Turnover Markers 128

Table 8.1 Dietary Reference Intakes for
Calcium and Vitamin D..150

Table 8.2 Sources of Vitamin D_2 and Vitamin D_3 166

Table 9.1 Agents Approved for the Treatment or
Prevention of Postmenopausal Osteoporosis 180

Table 9.2 Reduction in the Risk of Fractures and
All-Cause Mortality With Zoledronic Acid.........201

Table 9.3 Effect of Denosumab Compared With Placebo
on the Risk of Fractures at 36 Months 218

Table 9.4 Fracture Prevention Trial: Percent Changes
From Baseline in BMD With Teriparatide 236

FIGURES

Figure 1.1   Burden of Diseases in Europe Estimated as
              Disability-Adjusted Life-Years (DALYs)
              Lost Due to Osteoporosis and a Selection
              of Noncommunicable Diseases 12

Figure 1.2   Prevalence of Low Bone Mass and
              Osteoporosis in Women Aged 50 and Older
              in the United States 13

Figure 2.1   Bone Compartments and Those Principal
              Sites of Osteoporotic Fractures 20

Figure 2.2   Corticol Bone Envelopes or Surfaces 21

Figure 2.3   Type of Bone Loss With Age:
              A Comparison of Men and Women.......................24

Figure 2.4   Changes in Trabecular Bone Structure and
              Biomechanical Competence With Age..................25

Figure 2.5   Schematic Representation of Osteoclast
              Differentiation Supported by Osteoblasts/
              Stromal Cells...27

Figure 2.6   Schematic Drawing of Osteoclast Stimulators
              and Inhibitors 28

Figure 2.7   Signals That Determine Osteoblast
              Differentiation and Enhance Bone Formation 29

Figure 2.8   The Canonical Wnt/β-Catenin Signaling
              Pathway in Osteoblasts 30

Figure 2.9   Schematic Drawing of Osteoblast Stimulators
              and Inhibitors 32

Figure 2.10   Schematic Drawing Showing Overall
              Sequence of the Bone Remodeling Cycle.............33

Figure 3.1   Trabecular Bone Loss in Men vs Women 45

Figure 3.2   The Genesis of Hip Fractures in Older Women 46

Figure 3.3   Speed of Walking and the Direction of Falls 52

Figure 4.1   Fracture Risk Assessment Tool: FRAX® 69

Figure 4.2   Assessing Leg-Length Discrepancies 76

Figure 5.1   Prevalent Vertebral Fractures Increases
              Future Fracture Risk..85

Figure 5.2   Lumbar Spine DXA Scan..92

Figure 5.3   DXA Scan of the Hip 94

Figure 5.4   DXA Scan of the Wrist...96

Figure 5.5   Example of a DXA Facility Patient
             Questionnaire 98

Figure 5.6   Schematic Diagram of the Equipment Used
             for Ultrasonic Measurements 111

Figure 5.7   Quantitative Computerized Tomography for
             the Assessment of the Skeleton 113

Figure 5.8   Vertebral Fracture Assessment (VFA).................116

Figure 5.9   Schematic Diagram of a Semiquantitative
             Grading Scale for Vertebral Fractures.................120

Figure 5.10 The Trabecular Bone Score...................................122

Figure 6.1   Generation of BTMs During Type 1 Collagen
             Synthesis and Bone Resorption...........................130

Figure 7.1   Hip Protectors Attenuate Fracture Risk...............142

Figure 7.2   Vertebroplasty: Vertebral Compression
             Fracture Treatment Options.................................144

Figure 7.3   Kyphoplasty for Vertebral Compression.............145

Figure 8.1   Calcium Calculator...152

Figure 8.2   Interpretation of Food Labels for
             Calcium and Vitamin D Content 157

Figure 8.3   Vitamin D and Calcium Reduce Fracture Risk...159

Figure 8.4   Vitamin D, Calcium Absorption, and
             Bone Health...164

Figure 8.5   800 IU Oral Vitamin D_3 Reduces Risk for
             Osteoporotic Fractures 170

Figure 8.6   Direct and Indirect Effects of
             Vitamin D on Muscle 172

Figure 9.1   Bisphosphonates: Chemistry................................184

Figure 9.2   Bisphosphonate Cellular and Molecular
             Mechanisms of Action...186

Figure 9.3   Comparison of Change From Baseline to
12 Months in Hip Trochanter, Total Hip,
Femoral Neck, and Lumbar Spine BMD
in Once-Weekly Treatment With
Alendronate or Risedronate..................................188

Figure 9.4   Fracture Risk Reduction Comparing
5 Years (Alendronate/Placebo) vs 10 Years of
Alendronate (5 mg/10 mg) in the
Fracture Intervention Trials Long-Term
Extension (FLEX) Study.....................................190

Figure 9.5   Meta-analysis Comparing Fracture Risk
Reduction Due to Alendronate and Risedronate
in PMO and GIOP..192

Figure 9.6   Mean Change From Baseline in Lumbar Spine
and Hip BMD After 2 Years of Treatment With
Once-Monthly or Once-Daily Ibandronate.........197

Figure 9.7   Incidence of Morphometric Vertebral Fracture
With Once-Yearly IV Zoledronic Acid or
Placebo..200

Figure 9.8   Osteonecrosis of the Palatal Torus in a Patient
With Osteoporosis Taking Alendronate...............205

Figure 9.9   Atypical Femoral Subtrochanteric Fracture
and Prodromal Stress Fracture in a Patient
Who Received a Bisphosphonate.........................208

Figure 9.10 Mechanism of Action of RANKL Inhibitor
Denosumab...216

Figure 9.11 Cumulative Incidence of New Vertebral
Fractures in 7868 Postmenopausal Women
at Risk of Fracture During 36 Months of
Treatment With Denosumab or Placebo..............217

Figure 9.12 DATA-Switch: Mean Percent Change in
BMD From Baseline to 48 Months.....................222

Figure 9.13 DATA-Follow-Up: Percent Change in BMD
in Patients Who Did or Did Not Receive
Consolidation Therapy..224

Figure 9.14 DATA-Follow-Up: Percent Change in BMD
in Untreated Patients Who Discontinued
Teriparatide vs Denosumab at the End of
DATA-Switch..226

Figure 9.15 Results of the WHI Showing Comparative
Risks and Benefits of Combined Estrogen
and Progestin Compared With Placebo..............232

Figure 9.16 Fracture Prevention Trial: Teriparatide
Effect on Vertebral Fractures..............................236

Figure 9.17 ACTIVExtend: Incidence of Vertebral and
Nonvertebral Fractures..240

Figure 9.18 ACTIVE Trial: Kaplan-Meier Curve of
Time to First Incident Nonvertebral
Fractures by Treatment Group
(ITT Population)..241

Figure 9.19 Comparative Blunting of BMD and
Alkaline Phosphatase Using a Combination
of Alendronate and PTH(1-34) in
Bisphosphonate-Naïve Patients...........................242

Figure 9.20 Synergistic Effects on Lumbar Spine BMD of a
Combination of Zoledronic Acid and Teriparatide
Compared With Either Agent Alone 243

Figure 9.21 PTH Increased Trabecular Connectivity
and Cortical Wall Thickness................................245

Figure 10.1 Osteoclast Physiology and
Potential Therapeutic Targets..............................260

Figure 10.2 Osteoblast Physiology and
Potential Therapeutic Targets..............................263

Figure 11.1 PTH and Bone Turnover in CKD.......................272

Figure 11.2 The Pathophysiology of GIOP...........................275

Figure 11.3 ACR Guidelines: Initial Fracture Risk
Assessment..277

Figure 11.4 ACR Guidelines: Reassessment of
Fracture Risk 278

Figure 11.5 ACR Guidelines: Initial Pharmacologic
Treatment for Adults 282

Figure 11.6 BMD Loss With Cancer Therapies 284

1

Introduction: The Societal Burden of Osteoporosis

Osteoporosis is a systemic skeletal disease characterized by low bone mass and microarchitectural deterioration of bone tissue, with a consequent increase in bone fragility and the risk of fracture. Osteoporosis can affect both men and women, but white and Asian women, especially those who are past menopause, are at highest risk. Osteoporotic fractures are a significant cause of morbidity in older adults.

Hip fractures cause acute pain and loss of function, and nearly always lead to hospitalization. Recovery is slow and rehabilitation is often incomplete, with many patients permanently institutionalized in nursing homes. Vertebral fractures may cause acute pain and loss of function but may also occur without serious symptoms. However, vertebral fractures often recur, resulting in increased disability. Vertebral fractures also predict a significantly increased risk of fractures at other sites. Distal radius fractures also lead to acute pain and loss of function, but recovery of function is usually good or excellent. Furthermore, it is widely recognized that hip and vertebral fractures are associated with increased mortality. In the case of hip fracture, most deaths occur in the first 6 months following the event, of which 20% to 30% are causally related to the fracture event itself.

The individual and societal impact of osteoporosis has been assessed by comparing its associated burden of disability with other common noncommunicable diseases using Disability and Life-Years (DALYs) lost, which include deaths due to the disorder as well as the consequent disability in survivors. **Figure 1.1** shows the burden of osteoporosis in Europe expressed as DALYs compared with those for other chronic diseases. For example, osteoporosis accounted for

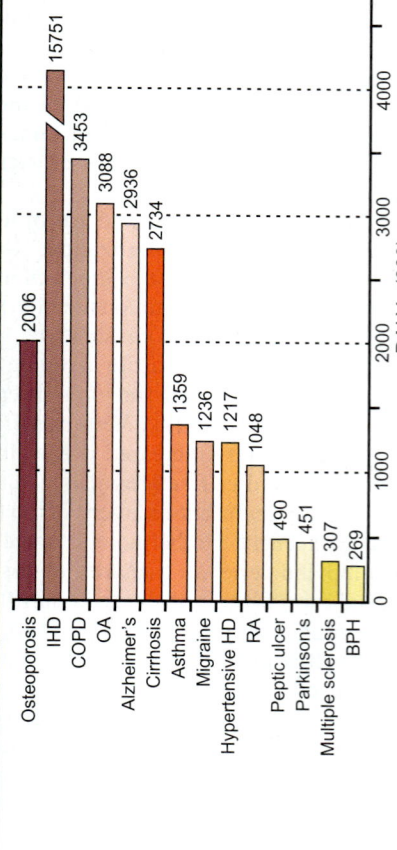

FIGURE 1.1 — Burden of Diseases in Europe Estimated as Disability-Adjusted Life-Years (DALYs) Lost Due to Osteoporosis and a Selection of Noncommunicable Diseases

Kanis JA, et al; European Society for Clinical and Economic Aspects of Osteoporosis and Osteoarthritis (ESCEO). *Osteoporos Int.* 2008; 19(4):399-428.

more DALYs than rheumatoid arthritis but fewer than osteoarthritis. Although not shown here, the burden of osteoporosis was greater than for all sites of cancer, with the exception of lung cancers. According to estimates from the US National Osteoporosis Foundation and the International Osteoporosis Foundation, the total annual direct costs resulting from osteoporotic fractures in 2012 was $19 billion in the United States alone and is expected to increase to over $25 billion in the US and $177 billion worldwide by 2025, on the basis of expected demographic changes and the burden of osteoporosis and its prodromal state, low bone mass (osteopenia) (**Figure 1.2**).

These high societal and personal costs of osteoporosis pose challenges to affected individuals, public health, and the medical community, particularly since most patients with osteoporosis remain untreated, and there has been a recent decline in the use of bone specific medications associated with societal percep-

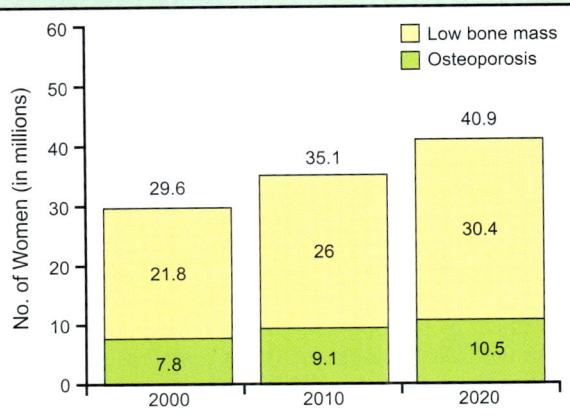

FIGURE 1.2 — Prevalence of Low Bone Mass and Osteoporosis in Women Aged 50 and Older in the United States

National Osteoporosis Foundation, personal communication, 2013.

tions of reduced benefit to risk. Furthermore, in light of increasing longevity, the prevalence of osteoporosis is rising, further adding to the current personal and societal burden.

Because bone loss occurs insidiously and is asymptomatic, osteoporosis often is diagnosed only after the first clinical fracture has occurred. Early assessment of an individual's risk of osteoporosis and subsequent fractures is therefore important to prevent the first fracture. International and country-specific guidelines have been proposed and/or implemented to address the challenge of screening for osteoporosis in an evidence-based and cost-effective manner. The determination of bone mineral density (BMD), as measured by dual-energy x-ray absorptiometry (DXA), is an established method to diagnose osteoporosis and to predict the risk of fracture (see *Chapter 5*).

In addition to low BMD, a number of other factors, such as age, low body mass index (BMI), previous fragility fractures, a family history of hip fractures, the use of glucocorticoids, cigarette smoking, and excessive alcohol consumption, can contribute to an individual's risk of future osteoporotic fractures. The role of non-BMD factors has been addressed in a new fracture risk assessment tool (FRAX) that can be used to estimate 10-year absolute risk for major osteoporotic and hip fracture probabilities from multiple clinical risk factors with or without hip BMD (see *Chapter 4*). The recent focus on the multiple pathologic and risk factors that influence fracture risk allows a highly individual-ized approach in the management of patients with osteoporosis beyond the exclusive reliance on BMD measurement.

The armamentarium of options for pharmacologic treatment of osteoporosis has increased considerably over the past few decades (see *Chapter 9*). Available anti-osteoporosis medications have unequivocally demonstrated their ability to reduce fractures at the spine significantly and, for most of them, at nonverte-bral skeletal sites. This has been achieved along with a reasonable safety profile, which brings the overall risk/benefit ratio of these medications into the upper range of what is usually seen in the management of chronic disorders. However, it is important to remember that the efficacy of present agents has only been demonstrated when used concurrently with adequate calcium and vitamin D supplementation.

New questions have emerged about the long-term safety of the most commonly used anti-osteoporosis medications, the bisphosphonates. During the past decade, there has been increasing understanding of bone biology, its molecular factors, the communication between bone-forming osteoblasts and bone-resorbing osteoclasts, and the orchestrating signaling networks (see *Chapter 2*). This has led to the identification of new therapeutic targets and the development of novel antiresorptive and anabolic agents (see *Chapter 10*).

Given the serious health and economic implications of osteoporotic fractures, it is essential to invest resources for the prevention of osteoporosis-associated fractures. This can be achieved by minimizing or eliminating factors that may contribute to loss of bone mass and risk of fractures, such as:

- Educating the lay community about the importance of developing and maintaining maximal bone mass
- Lifestyle modifications (cessation of smoking, reduction of alcohol consumption, increased physical activity) (see *Chapter 7*)
- Vitamin D and calcium supplementation (see *Chapter 8*)
- Fall prevention (see *Chapters 3* and *7*).

The efficacy of these measures can be aided by instituting them as early as possible, with the goal of maximizing bone mass as early as possible, and continuing them with the goal of minimizing the inevitable loss of bone mass over time.

All health care providers, including primary care physicians, obstetricians, and gynecologists, nurse practitioners, and physician assistants, can play pivotal roles in recognizing individuals at risk for osteoporosis and fractures, and educating those patients regarding measures to maintain bone health. Included also are allied health care professionals such as nutritionists, exercise science specialists, physical therapists, and pharmacists.

We hope this handbook will provide the information useful to the practitioner for understanding osteoporosis and its application for its prevention and treatment.

SUGGESTED READING

Body JJ, Bergmann P, Boonen S, et al. Evidence-based guidelines for the pharmacological treatment of postmenopausal osteoporosis: a consensus document by the Belgian Bone Club. *Osteoporos Int.* 2010;21(10):1657-1680.

Johnell O, Kanis JA. An estimate of the worldwide prevalence and disability associated with osteoporotic fractures. *Osteoporos Int.* 2006;17(12):1726-1733.

Kanis JA, Burlet N, Cooper C, et al; European Society for Clinical and Economic Aspects of Osteoporosis and Osteoarthritis (ESCEO). European guidance for the diagnosis and management of osteoporosis in postmenopausal women. *Osteoporos Int.* 2008;19(4):399-428.

Lecart MP, Reginstert JV. Current options for the management of postmenopausal osteoporosis. *Expert Opin Pharmacother.* 2011; 12(16):2533-2552.

Leslie WD, Schousboe JT. A review of osteoporosis diagnosis and treatment options in new and recently updated guidelines on case finding around the world. *Curr Osteoporos Rep.* 2011;9(3):129-140.

Nelson HD, Haney EM, Dana T, Bougatsos C, Chou R. Screening for osteoporosis: an update for the U.S. Preventive Services Task Force. *Ann Intern Med.* 2010;153(2):99-111.

North American Menopause Society. Management of osteoporosis in postmenopausal women: 2010 position statement. *Menopause.* 2010;17(1):25-54.

Rachner TD, Khosla S, Hofbauer LC. Osteoporosis: now and the future. *Lancet.* 2011;377(9773):1276-1287.

Siris ES, Selby PL, Saag KG, Borgstrom F, Herings RM, Silverman SL. Impact of osteoporosis treatment adherence on fracture rates in North America and Europe. *Am J Med.* 2009;122(suppl 2):S3-S13.

US Preventive Services Task Force. Screening for osteoporosis: U.S. Preventive Task Force Recommendation Statement. *Ann Intern Med.* 2011;154(5):356-364.

1

2　The Physiology of Bone

Bone Structure

Bone is a dynamic living tissue. The skeleton serves four important functions:
- Scaffold for the musculoskeletal system
- Protection of vital internal organs
- Reservoir of calcium and phosphorus
- Compartment for hematopoiesis

■ **Embryological Structure**
- *Intramembranous bone*: Bone arising from the ossification of mesenchymal cell condensations that occurs during embryological development. Examples include the flat bones of the skull, maxilla, mandible, pelvis, and clavicles.
- *Endochondral bone*: Bone arising when osteoblasts invade a preformed cartilaginous backbone. The continual growth and expansion of a cartilaginous band that is followed by osteoblast invasion constitutes the epiphyseal growth plate. This process ceases with puberty. Examples include all long bones and the spine.

■ **Anatomical Structure**
- *Axial skeleton*: The skull, spine, sacrum, sternum, and ribs comprise the axial skeleton (**Figure 2**.**1**).
- *Appendicular skeleton*: The clavicles, scapulae, pelvis, and the bones of the arms and legs comprise the appendicular skeleton (**Figure 2**.**1**).

■ **Architectural Structure**
- *Cortical bone*: is the dense outer shell of that has three surfaces (**Figure 2**.**2**). Each has different anatomic features but similar cell types and a similar bone remodeling cycle. The three surfaces are:

FIGURE 2.1 — Bone Compartments and Those Principal Sites of Osteoporotic Fractures

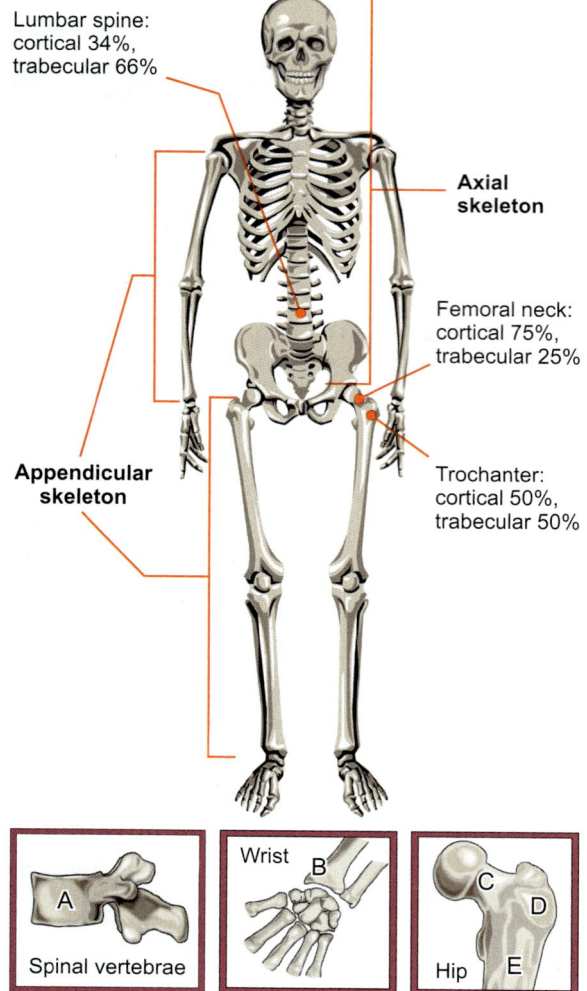

Lumbar spine: cortical 34%, trabecular 66%

Axial skeleton

Femoral neck: cortical 75%, trabecular 25%

Appendicular skeleton

Trochanter: cortical 50%, trabecular 50%

A — Spinal vertebrae

Wrist — B

Hip — C, D, E

Fractures of the spinal vertebrae, the wrist, and the hip are the most common, although other types of fractures also occur in individuals with osteoporosis.

FIGURE 2.2 — Cortical Bone Envelopes or Surfaces

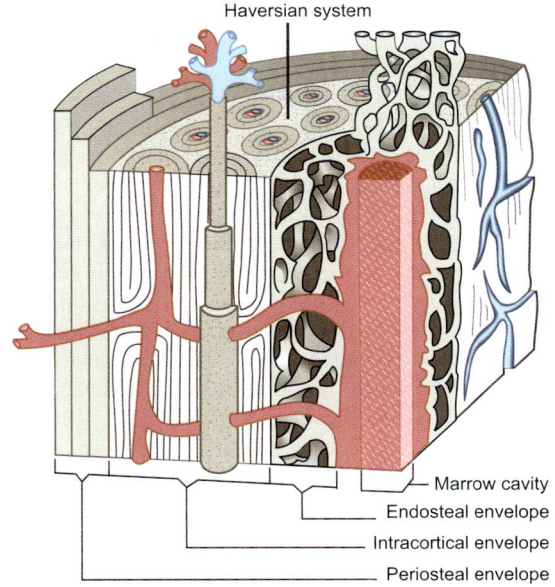

Haversian system

Marrow cavity
Endosteal envelope
Intracortical envelope
Periosteal envelope

- – Endosteum: The surface facing the marrow cavity
- – Periosteum: The outer surface of the bone
- – Intracortical bone: Bony space between the endosteum and periosteum

Within cortical bone lies the Haversian system (**Figure 2.2**). Concentric layers of lamellar bone are arranged around a central canal containing blood vessels and nerve fibers (also known as cortical osteons). These structures are the remnants of channels excavated by osteoclasts through cortical bone followed by the filling of these channels by bone-forming osteoblasts.

- *Trabecular bone*: This type of bone, also known as cancellous or spongy bone, is surrounded by cortical bone and has a honeycomb-like arrangement of interconnected plates. The plates are connected by rods and collectively provide additional strength to bone. Trabecular bone provides a framework for blood vessels and a foundation for hematopoietic cell production.

The bones of the axial and appendicular skeleton contain both cortical and trabecular bone, but the axial skeleton is predominantly composed of trabecular bone and the appendicular skeleton has a larger cortical component. One particular bone will often have different proportions of trabecular and cortical bone. At the ends of the long bones, there are variable regional combinations of trabecular and cortical bone. For example, vertebral bodies are comprised mostly of trabecular bone (**Figure 2**.1-**A**). The ultradistal radius (1.5 cm proximal to the styloid process) consists of approximately 25% cortical bone and 75% trabecular bone (**Figure 2**.1-**B**); whereas the 1/3 radius (measured at one third the length of the radius from the styloid process) is mainly cortical bone. A similar variable composition is noted in the femoral neck (**Figure 2**.1-**C**), the greater trochanter (**Figure 2**.1-**D**), and the shaft of the femur (**Figure 2**.1-**E**). Of note, healthy trabecular bone is designed to withstand compressive loads, while non-osteoporotic cortical bone provides support for torsional forces.

- ■ **Chemical Structure**
    - • *Collagenous proteins*: Type I collagen is the most prominent collagen in humans.[1] It is composed of a triple helix containing two identical $\alpha1(I)$ changes and a single $\alpha2(I)$ chain, both of which are encoded by two separate genes. Other important bone collagens include type III and V that assist in collagen assembly and fibril diameter.[2-4]
    - • *Non-collagenous proteins*: Non-collagenous proteins collectively regulate collagen fibril organization and the precipitation of hydroxy-

apatite crystals onto collagen fibrils.[5] Examples include osteocalcin, osteopontin, bone sialoprotein, and alkaline phosphatase.

- *Hydroxyapatite*: The combination of collagenous and non-collagenous proteins creates an environment for optimal precipitation, crystallization, and deposition of calcium and phosphorus onto the skeletal matrix. Hydroxyapatite is the mineral phase of bone with the molecular formula of $Ca_{10}(PO_4)_6(OH)_2$.

Bone Remodeling

Bone is a dynamic tissue undergoing continuous resorption and formation.[6] As with any architectural structure subjected to constant stress and strain, damage, such as fractures and microcracks, is repaired to restore structural integrity. Bone remodeling also mobilizes calcium and phosphorus from bone to maintain normal circulating levels of these minerals. Bone remodeling occurs predominantly within the large surface area of trabecular bone. The balance between bone resorption and bone formation determines whether net bone loss or bone formation occurs. Bone formation is greater than bone resorption until around age 30, the time of peak bone mass in men and women (**Figure 2.3**). During menopause and many other metabolic bone diseases, the balance tips toward resorption and bone loss. In the spine for example, excessive bone resorption results in thinning of trabecular plates, disappearance of trabecular rods, and loss of structural integrity (**Figure 2.4**).

The activity of the bone remodeling cycle varies depending on age and reproductive status.

- *Childhood*: New bone formation on the periosteum exceeds endosteal bone breakdown. The result is a net increase in the outer diameter of bone. The process of bone "modeling" occurs in childhood to create new bone mass during growth.

FIGURE 2.3 — Type of Bone Loss With Age: A Comparison of Men and Women

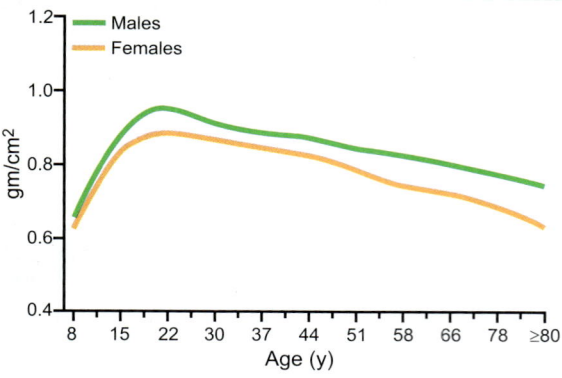

Looker AC, et al. National Center for Health Statistics. *Vital Health Stat.* 2012:11(251).

- *Adolescence*: Bone formation occurs on both the endosteal and periosteal surfaces with an increase in total bone mass. The process of bone "remodeling" occurs in adults that serves to repair older bone to restore architectural integrity.
- *Adulthood*: Endosteal bone loss increases and begins to exceed periosteal bone apposition, indicating the beginning of age- or menopause-related decrease in bone mass, with a resulting narrowing of the intracortical envelope. Expansion of the marrow cavity is a consequence.

Three types of cells regulate bone remodeling: osteoclasts, osteoblasts, and osteocytes.

■ **Osteoclasts**
Osteoclasts are specialized, multinucleated cells derived from the hematopoietic lineage. The main function of osteoclasts is resorption of mineralized

FIGURE 2.4 — Changes in Trabecular Bone Structure and Biomechanical Competence With Age

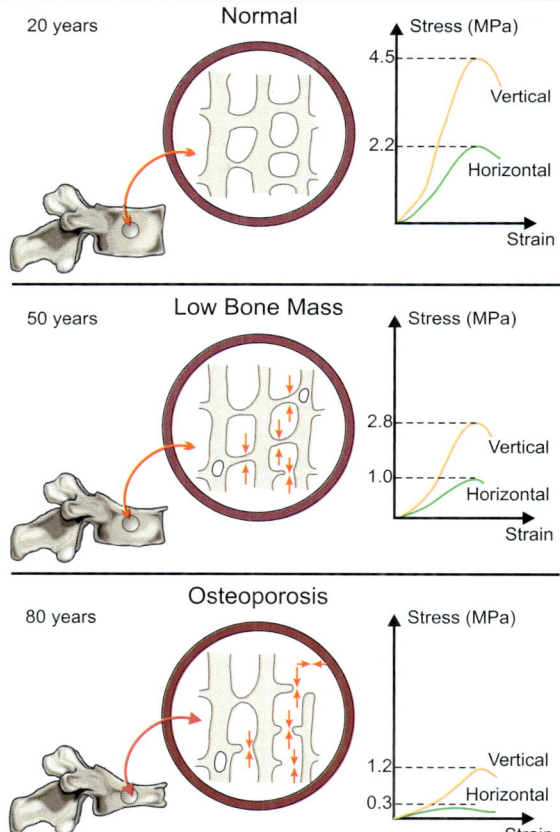

Changes in trabecular architecture and concomitant alterations in compressive strength of vertebrae with increasing age. Notice the initial preferential loss of horizontal trabeculae.

Modified from Takahashi HE, ed. *Bone Morphometry*. London, England: Nishimura/Smith Gordon, Niigata; 1990:367-370.

bone. Osteoclast differentiation is regulated by M-CSF and the receptor activator of NF-κB ligand (RANK-ligand [RANKL]) produced by cells of the osteoblast lineage including osteocytes (**Figure 2.5**).[7-10] Binding of RANKL to its receptor (RANK) present on pre-osteoclasts stimulates differentiation and inhibits apoptosis.[8,11,12] Osteoblasts also express a secreted factor called osteoprotegerin (OPG), which operates as a decoy receptor for RANKL.[13] By binding RANKL, it prevents binding to RANK on pre-osteoclasts and blocks osteoclastogenesis. Therefore, the ratio of RANKL:OPG determines the extent of bone resorption. The important regulator of bone resorption is parathyroid hormone (PTH). Although the PTH receptor is located on cells of the osteoblast lineage, PTH acts to increase the RANKL:OPG ratio.[14]

Other factors influencing RANKL:OPG include $1\alpha,25(OH)_2D_3$, the active form of vitamin D (**Figure 2.5**). In addition to the RANKL system, differentiation and activation of pre-osteoclasts to mature osteoclasts is influenced by numerous hormonal and growth factors (**Figure 2.6**).[7] For example, tumor necrosis factor-α, and interleukin-1 act as inflammatory cytokines, and the increase of these factors may be responsible for enhanced bone resorption and accelerated bone loss seen in inflammatory conditions such as rheumatoid arthritis and inflammatory bowel diseases.[15]

The characteristic feature of a fully differentiated and activated osteoclast is a ruffled border enclosing a sealing zone over the site of active resorption. Once the area below the osteoclast is sealed and isolated from the surrounding environment, protons are secreted creating a highly acidic environment with a pH of 3-4 that dissolves hydroxyapatite. Hydrolytic enzymes, namely cathepsin K and matrix metalloproteinases, cooperate with the acidic microenvironment to degrade the protein phase of the bone matrix.[16]

■ **Osteoblasts**

Osteoblasts are derived from mesenchymal stem cells and are responsible for bone matrix synthesis

FIGURE 2.5 — Schematic Representation of Osteoclast Differentiation Supported by Osteoblasts/Stromal Cells

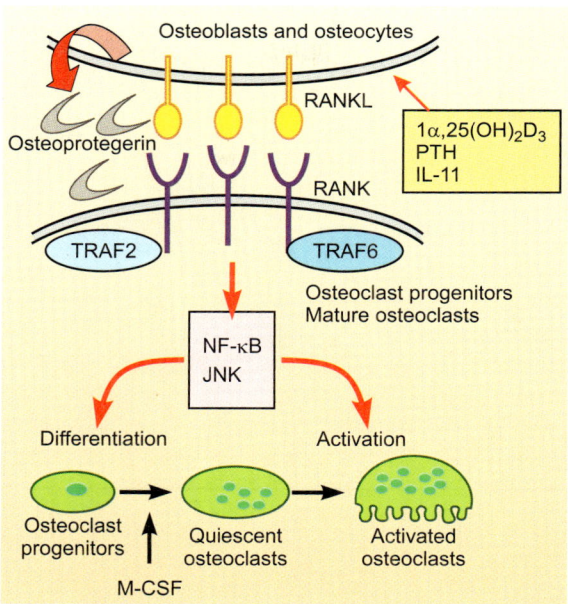

RANKL, which is induced by bone resorbing factors such as $1\alpha,25(OH)_2D_3$, parathyroid hormone (PTH), and IL-11 on the plasma membrane of osteoblasts/stromal cells, binds its receptor RANK present in osteoclast progenitors and mature osteoclasts. Osteoprotegerin (OPG), a decoy receptor for RANKL, strongly and competitively inhibits the RANKL–RANK interaction. The RANK signaling is transduced via TNF receptor-associated factor 2 (TRAF2) and TNF receptor-associated factor 6 (TRAF6), leading to the activation of NF-κB and Jun kinase (JNK), which in turn stimulates differentiation and activation of osteoclasts. M-CSF, macrophage colony-stimulating factor.

Udagawa N, et al. *Arthritis Res*. 2002;4(5):281-289.

FIGURE 2.6 — Schematic Drawing of Osteoclast Stimulators and Inhibitors

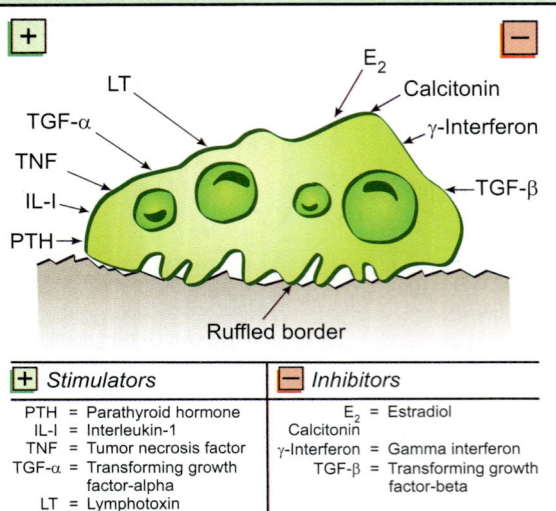

⊞ *Stimulators*	⊟ *Inhibitors*
PTH = Parathyroid hormone IL-I = Interleukin-1 TNF = Tumor necrosis factor TGF-α = Transforming growth factor-alpha LT = Lymphotoxin	E_2 = Estradiol Calcitonin γ-Interferon = Gamma interferon TGF-β = Transforming growth factor-beta

and its subsequent mineralization. Factors present in primordial bone include the bone morphogenetic proteins, Wnt (Wingless-type MMTV integration site) ligands, and Hedgehog proteins. These secreted factors regulate expression of the RUNX2 transcription factor in mesenchymal stem cells that direct pluripotent cells to an osteoblast fate (**Figure 2.7**).[17] Other osteoblast transcription factors that coordinate with RUNX2 to ensure proper osteoblast development include DLX3, DLX5, MSX2, and Osterix.[18-21] PTH enhances pre-osteoblast proliferation and differentiation. Bone formation by mature osteoblasts is enhanced by the synthesis of insulin-like growth factor 1, which is triggered by PTH and growth hormone.[22]

The Wnt family of ligands has critical effects throughout osteoblast development.[23] Wnt signaling uses the so-called canonical Wnt/β-catenin signaling pathway to regulate osteoblast gene expression (**Figure 2.8**). Wnt ligands bind to specific receptors, called

FIGURE 2.7 — Signals That Determine Osteoblast Differentiation and Enhance Bone Formation

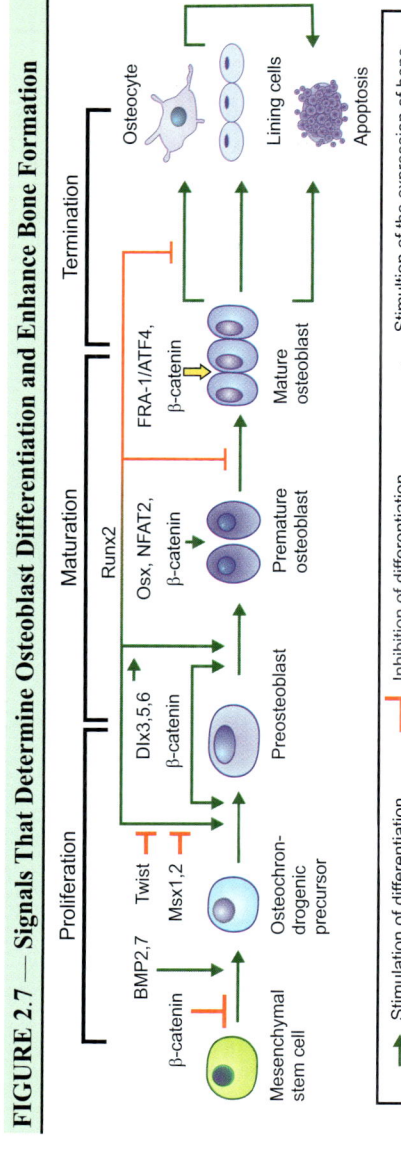

Undifferentiated mesenchymal cells differentiate toward cells of the osteoblastic lineage under the influence of multiple signaling pathways.

Rosen CJ, et al, ed. *Primer on the Metabolic Bone Disease and Disorders of Mineral Metabolism.* 7th ed. Hoboken, NJ: Wiley, Inc; 2008.

2

FIGURE 2.8 — The Canonical Wnt/β-Catenin Signaling Pathway in Osteoblasts

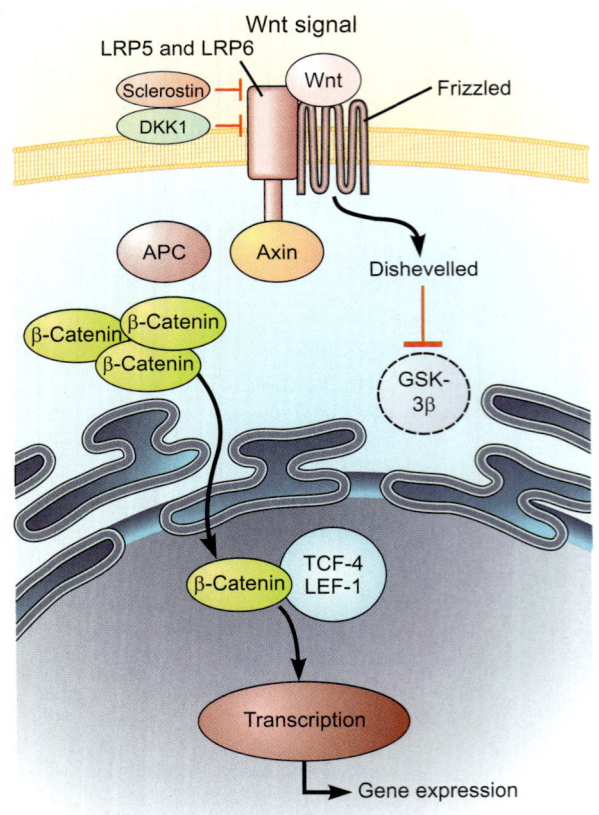

Wnt binding to its receptor (Frizzled) and coreceptors (low-density lipoprotein receptor–related proteins 5 and 6 [LRP5 and LRP6]), induces Dishevelled, an intracellular protein that degrades glycogen synthase kinase 3 β (GSK-3β). These two events lead to the stabilization of β-catenin and its translocation to the nucleus and ultimately, gene expression. Secreted Wnt antagonists that interact with Wnt coreceptors LRP-5/6 include sclerostin and Dickkopf (Dkk-1) and sclerostin,

Adapted from Canalis E, et al. *N Engl J Med.* 2007;357:905-916.

Frizzled. Low-density lipoprotein receptor–related proteins 5 and 6 (LRP5 and LRP6) act as co-receptors for Frizzled to bind Wnt.[24-26] These interactions lead to the stabilization of intracytoplasmic β-catenin, which translocates to the nucleus and regulates gene expression. This bone-anabolic pathway appears to be principally regulated by Wnt inhibitors, such as Dickkopf-1 (DKK1) and Sclerostin, which bind and block the Wnt receptor LRP5 and LRP6.[27-29] These Wnt inhibitors serve as targets for emerging novel agents that enhance bone formation.

In addition to the above mechanisms, osteoblasts are also influenced by numerous other hormonal and growth factors (**Figure 2.9**).

■ Osteocytes

These cells are derived from osteoblasts that become encased within the newly formed osteoid after the bone formation phase is completed.[30] Osteocytes situated deep in bone matrix maintain contact with newly incorporated osteocytes in osteoid, and with osteoblasts and bone lining cells on the bone surfaces, through an extensive network of cell processes (canaliculi). Osteocytes sense mechanical strain of bone, respond to bone damage (eg, microcracks), and transmit messages to the bone lining cells (the resting phase of osteoblasts), directing them to initiate the bone remodeling cycle.[31] This process also recruits an assembly of cells (osteoclasts and osteoblasts) into a discrete temporary anatomic structure called a basic multicellular unit (BMU), which performs all of the processes required for bone repair and remodeling.[32] Osteocytes exclusively produce and secrete sclerostin, an inhibitor of the Wnt-signaling pathway, which inhibits osteoblast differentiation and bone formation.[33,34] Osteocytes also express fibroblast growth factor-23 (FGF-23), an endocrine hormone that regulates renal phosphate metabolism.[35,36]

■ The Bone Remodeling Cycle

The bone remodeling cycle consists of a number of sequential and interconnected steps, which under

FIGURE 2.9 — Schematic Drawing of Osteoblast Stimulators and Inhibitors

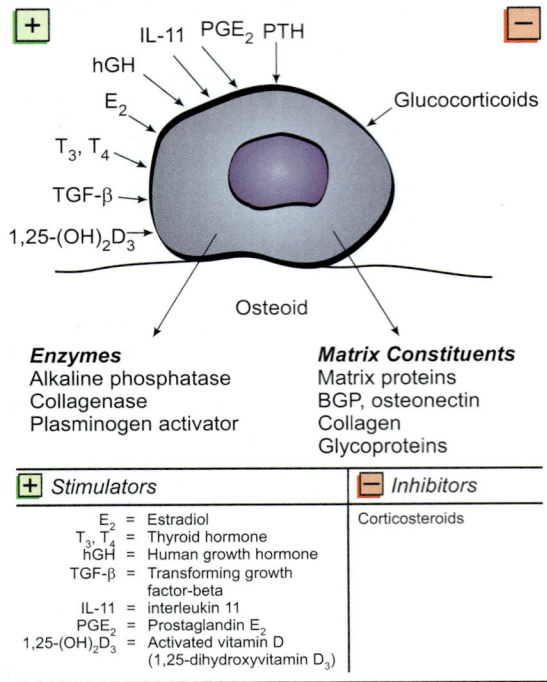

+ Stimulators		− Inhibitors
E_2 = Estradiol T_3, T_4 = Thyroid hormone hGH = Human growth hormone TGF-β = Transforming growth factor-beta IL-11 = interleukin 11 PGE_2 = Prostaglandin E_2 $1,25\text{-}(OH)_2D_3$ = Activated vitamin D $(1,25\text{-dihydroxyvitamin } D_3)$		Corticosteroids

normal circumstances, ensure that there is a balance between the amount of bone resorbed and the amount replaced.[6] This process involves crosstalk and signaling between the main bone cells and the extracellular environment. The overall sequence of the bone remodeling cycle is illustrated in **Figure 2.10**:

- *Activation:* As noted previously, remodeling is initiated by damage to bone which triggers programmed cell death (apoptosis) of local matrix-embedded osteocytes which, in turn, signal the location of damage and also recruit an assembly of cells (osteoclasts and osteoblasts) into a discrete temporary anatomic structure

FIGURE 2.10 — Schematic Drawing Showing Overall Sequence of the Bone Remodeling Cycle

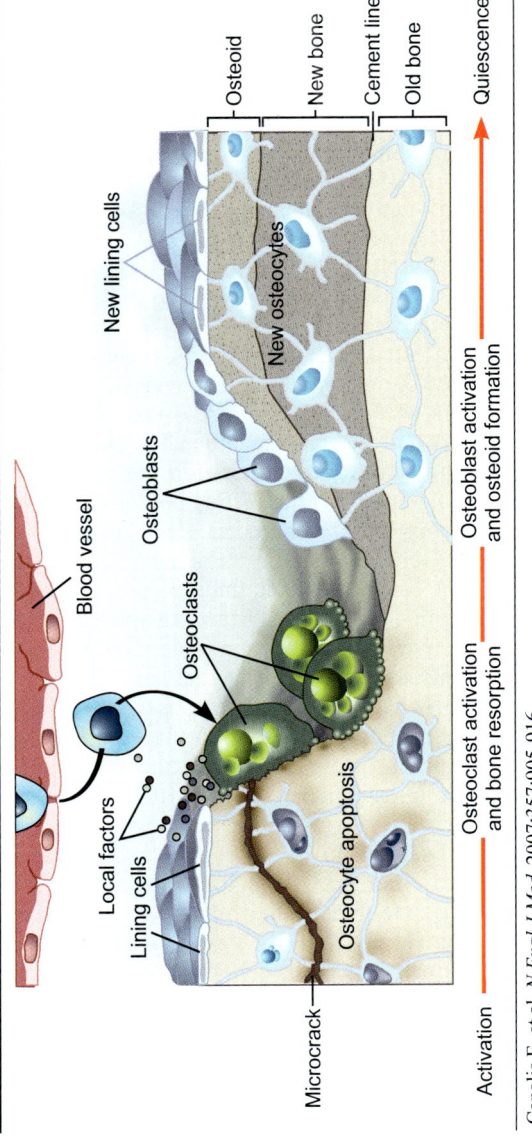

Canalis E, et al. *N Engl J Med.* 2007;357:905-916.

(BMU), which performs all of the processes required for bone repair and remodeling.

- *Osteoclast Activation and Resorption:* Stromal cells that have been activated by messages from osteocytes produce macrophage colony stimulating factor (M-CSF), which stimulates differentiation of cells into pre-osteoclasts. As noted previously, the differentiation of a fully activated osteoclast depends on the binding of osteocyte- and osteoblast-derived RANKL to RANK receptors on osteoclasts. Stromal cells also divide to produce pre-osteoblasts, which express RANKL on their cell surfaces. Pre-osteoclasts have RANK receptors on their surface. When RANKL activates RANK receptors on the surface of pre-osteoclasts, the cells fuse and differentiate into mature multinucleated osteoclasts, which develop the characteristic sealed zone with a ruffled border within which resorption of bone takes place. The resorption phase of remodeling lasts about 2 to 6 weeks. The osteoclasts then undergo programmed cell death or apoptosis. Osteoclast apoptosis may be delayed (and resorption prolonged) by estrogen deficiency and other factors.

- *Osteoblast Activation and Osteoid Formation:* As noted previously, recruitment and activation of osteoblasts is initiated through the Wnt/β-catenin pathway and RUNX2, the master switches for osteoblastic differentiation, and subsequently by other factors such as PTH and other growth factors. The active, secreting osteoblasts then make layers of osteoid and slowly refill the cavity. They also secrete growth factors, osteopontin, osteocalcin, OPG, and other proteins. When the osteoid is about 6 microns thick, it begins to mineralize. This process also is regulated by the osteocytes, which regulate phosphate metabolism. Estrogens and other hormones regulate osteoblast lifespan.

For months after the cavity has been filled with bone, the crystals of mineral are packed more closely and the density of the new bone increases.

- *Quiescence:* Some of the remaining osteoblasts become new bone lining cells that participate in the minute-to-minute release of calcium from the bones through bone resorption. Some of the osteoblasts also turn into new osteocytes that remain in the bone, connected by long cell processes that can sense mechanical stresses to the bone.

Systemic Endocrine Factors Influencing Bone Metabolism

The chief cells of the parathyroid gland secrete PTH. This 84 amino acid protein is secreted in response to declining serum calcium concentration.[37] PTH in turn increases serum calcium and operates in a classical endocrine feedback loop to maintain circulating calcium concentration between 8.4 and 10.2 mg/dL. PTH binds to the parathyroid hormone receptor that is expressed on cells of the osteoblast lineage and bone marrow stromal cells, activates expression of M-CSF and RANKL, and indirectly stimulates osteoclastic bone resorption.[38] An important nonskeletal action of PTH is to stimulate increased renal reabsorption of calcium, which, together with increased resorption to mobilize calcium from bone, restores physiologic serum calcium levels.[39] PTH also stimulates the production of the active metabolite of vitamin D, 1,25-dihydroxyvitamin D ($1,25(OH)_2D_3$), from its circulating inactive precursor 25-hydroxyvitamin D.[40] In turn, $1,25(OH)_2D_3$ facilitates calcium absorption from the gut and the kidney and positively regulates bone resorption indirectly through the vitamin D receptors in osteoblasts, which increases RANKL and M-CSF expression.[41]

The major role for estrogen in the skeletal system is as a bone-sparing hormone that acts through receptors expressed by both osteoclasts and osteoblasts.[42,43] This sex hormone is crucial in the control of osteoclast lifespan and can cause pre-osteoclast and osteoclast apoptosis.[44,45] Therefore, loss of estrogen in women after the menopause results in increased osteoclast formation and survival. Estrogen also blocks osteoclast function indirectly through effects on the immune system and has a role in regulating the response of bone to mechanical stimulation.[46-50]

Other hormones also have significant actions in bone homeostasis. Parafollicular cells (also known as C-cells) located within the thyroid gland secrete calcitonin.[51] Its secretion is stimulated by increased serum calcium concentration. Calcitonin has numerous actions including inhibiting osteoclastic bone resorption, intestinal calcium absorption, and renal calcium reabsorption. Although calcitonin was once thought to be a major regulator of bone homeostasis throughout life, it appears to have a more limited protective role to prevent excessive bone resorption during pregnancy and lactation.[52]

Hyperthyroidism is a risk factor for bone loss. Through overactivation of thyroid hormone receptors in osteoblasts and osteoclasts, excessive thyroid hormone leads to a net increase in bone resorption and increased fracture risk.[53-55] Similarly, osteoblasts and osteoclasts have glucocorticoid receptors. Excess glucocorticoid activity (or long-term glucocorticoid treatment) results in inhibition of osteoblastic bone formation and activation of osteoclastic bone resorption.[56,57] Glucocorticoids compound these direct negative effects on bone by decreasing intestinal calcium absorption and increasing renal calcium loss.[58-60]

Mechanical Stress and Force

Mechanical force (eg, physical exercise) is also a key regulator of bone remodeling and of bone architecture in general.[61,62] It influences bone metabolism not only locally, but also systemically (as illustrated by the profound bone loss in astronauts experiencing zero gravity and in immobilized patients). In vivo and in vitro studies have confirmed that osteocytes and osteoblasts are able to sense and respond to mechanical forces.[33,63,64] Early signals produced in response to mechanical stimuli include nitric oxide, prostaglandins, and Wnt signaling proteins. However, the precise mechanical stimulus that is sensed by bone cells in vivo and the signal produced as a result remain unclear.

REFERENCES

1. Viguet-Carrin S, Garnero P, Delmas PD. The role of collagen in bone strength. *Osteoporos Int*. 2006;17:319-336.

2. Superti-Furga A, Gugler E, Gitzelmann R, Steinmann B. Ehlers-Danlos syndrome type IV: a multi-exon deletion in one of the two COL3A1 alleles affecting structure, stability, and processing of type III procollagen. *J Biol Chem*. 1988;263: 6226-6232.

3. Wenstrup RJ, Florer JB, Brunskill EW, Bell SM, Chervoneva I, Birk DE. Type V collagen controls the initiation of collagen fibril assembly. *J Biol Chem*. 2004;279:53331-53337.

4. Weis MA, Hudson DM, Kim L, Scott M, Wu JJ, Eyre DR. Location of 3-hydroxyproline residues in collagen types I, II, III, and V/XI implies a role in fibril supramolecular assembly. *J Biol Chem*. 2010;285:2580-2590.

5. Young MF, Kerr JM, Ibaraki K, Heegaard AM, Robey PG. Structure, expression, and regulation of the major noncollagenous matrix proteins of bone. *Clin Orthop Relat Res*. 1992;281:275-294.

6. Martin TJ, Seeman E. Bone remodelling: its local regulation and the emergence of bone fragility. *Best Pract Res Clin Endocrinol Metab*. 2008;22:701-722.

7. Yasuda H, Shima N, Nakagawa N, et al. Osteoclast differentiation factor is a ligand for osteoprotegerin/osteoclastogenesis-inhibitory factor and is identical to TRANCE/RANKL. *Proc Natl Acad Sci USA*. 1998;95:3597-3602.

8. Lacey DL, Timms E, Tan HL, et al. Osteoprotegerin ligand is a cytokine that regulates osteoclast differentiation and activation. *Cell*. 1998;93:165-176.

9. Pixley FJ, Stanley ER. CSF-1 regulation of the wandering macrophage: complexity in action. *Trends Cell Biol*. 2004;14:628-638.

10. Xiong J, Onal M, Jilka RL, Weinstein RS, Manolagas SC, O'Brien CA. Matrix-embedded cells control osteoclast formation. *Nat Med*. 2011;17:1235-1241.

11. Anderson DM, Maraskovsky E, Billingsley WL, et al. A homologue of the TNF receptor and its ligand enhance T-cell growth and dendritic-cell function. *Nature*. 1997;390:175-179.

12. Lacey DL, Tan HL, Lu J, et al. Osteoprotegerin ligand modulates murine osteoclast survival in vitro and in vivo. *Am J Pathol*. 2000;157:435-448.

13. Simonet WS, Lacey DL, Dunstan CR, et al. Osteoprotegerin: a novel secreted protein involved in the regulation of bone density. *Cell*. 1997;89:309-319.

14. Huang JC, Sakata T, Pfleger LL, et al. PTH differentially regulates expression of RANKL and OPG. *J Bone Miner Res*. 2004;19:235-244.

15. Walsh NC, Crotti TN, Goldring SR, Gravallese EM. Rheumatic diseases: the effects of inflammation on bone. *Immunol Rev*. 2005;208:228-251.

16. Teitelbaum SL, Ross FP. Genetic regulation of osteoclast development and function. *Nat Rev Genet*. 2003;4(8):638-649.

17. Otto F, Thornell AP, Crompton T, et al. Cbfa1, a candidate gene for cleidocranial dysplasia syndrome, is essential for osteoblast differentiation and bone development. *Cell*. 1997;89:765-771.

18. Hassan MQ, Javed A, Morasso MI, et al. Dlx3 transcriptional regulation of osteoblast differentiation: temporal recruitment of Msx2, Dlx3, and Dlx5 homeodomain proteins to chromatin of the osteocalcin gene. *Mol Cell Biol*. 2004;24:9248-9261.

19. Miyama K, Yamada G, Yamamoto TS, et al. A BMP-inducible gene, dlx5, regulates osteoblast differentiation and mesoderm induction. *Dev Biol*. 1999;208(1):123-133.

20. Matsubara T, Kida K, Yamaguchi A, et al. BMP2 regulates Osterix through Msx2 and Runx2 during osteoblast differentiation. *J Biol Chem*. 2008;283(43):29119-29125.

21. Nakashima K, Zhou X, Kunkel G, et al. The novel zinc finger-containing transcription factor osterix is required for osteoblast differentiation and bone formation. *Cell*. 2002;108:17-29.

22. Bikle D, Adams J, Christakos S. Vitamin D: Production, metabolism, mechanism of action, and clinical requirements. In: Rosen CJ, ed. *Primer on the Metabolic Bone Diseases and Disorders of Mineral Metabolism*. 7th ed. Washington, DC: American Society for Bone and Mineral Research; 2008:141-149.

23. Baron R, Rawadi G. Targeting the Wnt/beta-catenin pathway to regulate bone formation in the adult skeleton. *Endocrinology*. 2007;148(6):2635-2643.

24. Gong Y, Slee RB, Fukai N, et al. LDL receptor-related protein 5 (LRP5) affects bone accrual and eye development. *Cell*. 2001;107:513-523.

25. Boyden LM, Mao J, Belsky J, et al. High bone density due to a mutation in LDL-receptor-related protein 5. *N Engl J Med*. 2002;346:1513-1521.

26. Little RD, Carulli JP, Del Mastro RG, et al. A mutation in the LDL receptor-related protein 5 gene results in the autosomal dominant high-bone-mass trait. *Am J Hum Genet*. 2002;70(1): 11-19.

27. Li J, Sarosi I, Morony SE, et al. Transgenic mice over-expressing Dkk1 in osteoblasts develop osteoporosis. *J Bone Miner Res*. 2004;19:S6.

28. Niida A, Hiroko T, Kasai M, et al. DKK1, a negative regulator of Wnt signaling, is a target of the beta-catenin/TCF pathway. *Oncogene*. 2004;23:8520-8526.

29. Li X, Zhang Y, Kang H, et al. Sclerostin binds to LRP5/6 and antagonizes canonical Wnt signaling. *J Biol Chem*. 2005;280: 19883-19887.

30. Franz-Odendaal TA, Hall BK, Witten PE. Buried alive: how osteoblasts become osteocytes. *Dev Dyn*. 2006;235(1):176-190.

31. Turner CH, Forwood MR, Otter MW. Mechanotransduction in bone: do bone cells act as sensors of fluid flow? *FASEB J*. 1994;8:875-878.

32. Hauge EM, Qvesel D, Eriksen EF, Mosekilde L, Melsen F. Cancellous bone remodeling occurs in specialized compartments lined by cells expressing osteoblastic markers. *J Bone Miner Res*. 2001;16(9):1575-1582.

33. Robling AG, Niziolek PJ, Baldridge LA, et al. Mechanical stimulation of bone in vivo reduces osteocyte expression of Sost/sclerostin. *J Biol Chem*. 2008;283:5866-5875.

34. Winkler DG, Sutherland MK, Geoghegan JC, et al. Osteocyte control of bone formation via sclerostin, a novel BMP antagonist. *EMBO J*. 2003;22:6267-6276.

35. ADHR C. Autosomal dominant hypophosphataemic rickets is associated with mutations in FGF23. *Nat Genet*. 2000;26:345-348.

36. Liu S, Zhou J, Tang W, Jiang X, Rowe DW, Quarles LD. Pathogenic role of Fgf23 in Hyp mice. *Am J Physiol Endocrinol Metab*. 2006;291:E38-E49.

37. Potts JT. Parathyroid hormone: past and present. *J Endocrinol*. 2005;187:311-325.

38. Murray TM, Rao LG, Divieti P, Bringhurst FR. Parathyroid hormone secretion and action: evidence for discrete receptors for the carboxyl-terminal region and related biological actions of carboxyl- terminal ligands. *Endocr Rev*. 2005;26(1):78-113.

39. van Abel M, Hoenderop JG, van der Kemp AW, Friedlaender MM, van Leeuwen JP, Bindels RJ. Coordinated control of renal

Ca(2+) transport proteins by parathyroid hormone. *Kidney Int.* 2005;68:1708-1721.

40. Broadus AE, Horst RL, Lang R, Littledike ET, Rasmussen H. The importance of circulating 1,25-dihydroxyvitamin D in the pathogenesis of hypercalciuria and renal-stone formation in primary hyperparathyroidism. *N Engl J Med.* 1980;302:421-426.

41. Raisz LG, Trummel CL, Holick MF, DeLuca HF. 1,25-dihydroxycholecalciferol: a potent stimulator of bone resorption in tissue culture. *Science.* 1972;175:768-769.

42. Hughes DE, Dai A, Tiffee JC, Li HH, Mundy GR, Boyce BF. Estrogen promotes apoptosis of murine osteoclasts mediated by TGF-beta. *Nat Med.* 1996;2:1132-1136.

43. Riggs BL. The mechanisms of estrogen regulation of bone resorption. *J Clin Invest.* 2000;106:1203-1204.

44. Shevde NK, Bendixen AC, Dienger KM, Pike JW. Estrogens suppress RANK ligand-induced osteoclast differentiation via a stromal cell independent mechanism involving c-Jun repression. *Proc Natl Acad Sci USA.* 2000;97:7829-7834.

45. Nakamura T, Imai Y, Matsumoto T, et al. Estrogen prevents bone loss via estrogen receptor alpha and induction of Fas ligand in osteoclasts. *Cell.* 2007;130:811-823.

46. Cenci S, Weitzmann MN, Roggia C, et al. Estrogen deficiency induces bone loss by enhancing T-cell production of TNF-alpha. *J Clin Invest.* 2000;106:1229-1237.

47. Cenci S, Toraldo G, Weitzmann MN, et al. Estrogen deficiency induces bone loss by increasing T cell proliferation and lifespan through IFN-gamma-induced class II transactivator. *Proc Natl Acad Sci USA.* 2003;100:10405-10410.

48. Ryan MR, Shepherd R, Leavey JK, et al. An IL-7-dependent rebound in thymic T cell output contributes to the bone loss induced by estrogen deficiency. *Proc Natl Acad Sci USA.* 2005;102:16735-16740.

49. Armstrong VJ, Muzylak M, Sunters A, et al. Wnt/beta-catenin signaling is a component of osteoblastic bone cell early responses to load-bearing and requires estrogen receptor alpha. *J Biol Chem.* 2007;282:20715-20727.

50. Aguirre JI, Plotkin LI, Gortazar AR, et al. A novel ligand-independent function of the estrogen receptor is essential for osteocyte and osteoblast mechanotransduction. *J Biol Chem.* 2007;282:25501-25508.

51. Copp DH, Cheney B. Calcitonin-a hormone from the parathyroid which lowers the calcium-level of the blood. *Nature.* 1962;193:381-382.

52. Woodrow JP, Sharpe CJ, Fudge NJ, Hoff AO, Gagel RF, Kovacs CS. Calcitonin plays a critical role in regulating skeletal mineral metabolism during lactation. *Endocrinology.* 2006;147:4010-4021.

53. Britto JM, Fenton AJ, Holloway WR, Nicholson GC. Osteoblasts mediate thyroid hormone stimulation of osteoclastic bone resorption. *Endocrinology.* 1994;134:169-176.

54. Baliram R, Sun L, Cao J, et al. Hyperthyroid-associated osteoporosis is exacerbated by the loss of TSH signaling. *J Clin Invest.* 2012;122:3737-3741.

55. Bauer DC, Ettinger B, Nevitt MC, Stone KL. Risk for fracture in women with low serum levels of thyroid-stimulating hormone. *Ann Intern Med.* 2001;134:561-568.

56. Canalis E, Bilezikian JP, Angeli A, Giustina A. Perspectives on glucocorticoid-induced osteoporosis. *Bone.* 2004;34:593-598.

57. Manolagas SC, Weinstein RS. New developments in the pathogenesis and treatment of steroid-induced osteoporosis. *J Bone Miner Res.* 1999;14:1061-1066.

58. Hahn TJ, Halstead LR, Baran DT. Effects off short term glucocorticoid administration on intestinal calcium absorption and circulating vitamin D metabolite concentrations in man. *J Clin Endocrinol Metab.* 1981;52:111-115.

59. Huybers S, Naber TH, Bindels RJ, Hoenderop JG. Prednisolone-induced Ca2+ malabsorption is caused by diminished expression of the epithelial Ca2+ channel TRPV6. *Am J Physiol Gastrointest Liver Physiol.* 2007;292:G92-G97.

60. Suzuki Y, Ichikawa Y, Saito E, Homma M. Importance of increased urinary calcium excretion in the development of secondary hyperparathyroidism of patients under glucocorticoid therapy. *Metabolism.* 1983;32:151-156.

61. Malone AM, Anderson CT, Tummala P, et al. Primary cilia mediate mechanosensing in bone cells by a calcium-independent mechanism. *Proc Natl Acad Sci USA.* 2007;104:13325-13330.

62. Ozcivici E, Luu YK, Adler B, et al. Mechanical signals as anabolic agents in bone. *Nat Rev Rheumatol.* 2010;6(1):50-59.

63. Patel MJ, Chang KH, Sykes MC, Talish R, Rubin C, Jo H. Low magnitude and high frequency mechanical loading prevents decreased bone formation responses of 2T3 preosteoblasts. *J Cell Biochem.* 2009;106:306-316.

64. Thompson WR, Rubin CT, Rubin J. Mechanical regulation of signaling pathways in bone. *Gene.* 2012;503:179-193.

3

Pathogenesis of Osteoporosis and Other Metabolic Bone Diseases

Clinical Types

■ Primary or Idiopathic Osteoporosis

Menopausal women with osteoporosis in whom no contributory underlying medical condition is present are said to have primary osteoporosis. Estrogen deficiency at menopause is responsible for this type of osteoporosis. For an American woman aged 50, the risk of having an osteoporotic fracture in the remainder of her life is 40%.[1] Bone turnover rate, particularly bone loss, accelerates 3 to 5 years before the last menstrual period and slows again 3 to 5 years after the last menstrual period.[2] During the menopausal transition, the mean rate of bone loss during this period is about 1% to 2% per year or about 10% during the entire period. This seemingly insignificant decline in bone mass in fact translates into a significant 2- to 3-fold greater fracture risk.[3]

■ Secondary Osteoporosis

Secondary forms of osteoporosis and metabolic disorders that result in low bone mass and fractures are discussed in *Chapter 4* and *Chapter 11*.

Pathogenesis

Important architectural changes occur with osteoporosis:

Trabecular bone thinning and damage results from:
- Increased activity of osteoclasts and resorption sites with pathologically deep resorptive cavities resulting in perforation of trabecular plates. The process is accelerated by resorption

at opposite sites of the same trabecula with one lacuna penetrating into another. Increased bone resorptive activity after menopause in women leads to perforation of the trabeculae (**Figure 3.1**).[4] Testosterone deficiency in older men also increases bone resorption but not to the degree of estrogen deficiency in women.[5] Such declines in testosterone that occurs with aging leads to trabecular thinning but the basic trabecular structure may be preserved (**Figure 3.1**).

- Decreased osteoblast activity causes impairment in the repair of resorption perforations (**Figure 3.1**). Sex steroids influence the capacity for osteoblast renewal and bone repair.[6]

Cortical bone loss may be due to the following:

- Excessive endosteal osteoclast resorptive activity resulting in thinning of the cortex and irreversible bone loss (**Figure 3.1**).[7]
- Increased activity of the intracortical bone remodeling units resulting in greater porosity of the cortex.[8] This type of bone loss is potentially reversible.

The imbalance between osteoclastic bone resorption and osteoblast bone formation (see *Chapter 2*) varies according to the skeletal site and the underlying etiology (**Figure 3.2**). Five main factors ultimately determine fracture risk:

- Failure to achieve peak bone mass
- Accelerated bone loss
- Inadequate bone formation
- Poor bone quality with irreversible damage to the microarchitecture of the bone
- Increased fall risk.

■ **Failure to Achieve Peak Bone Mass**

Bone mass in the elderly, when the risk of fracture is highest, is dependent on the peak bone mass that was achieved in youth.[9-11] After about age 30, bone mass begins a slow decline. Therefore, strategies to

FIGURE 3.1 — Trabecular Bone Loss in Men vs Women

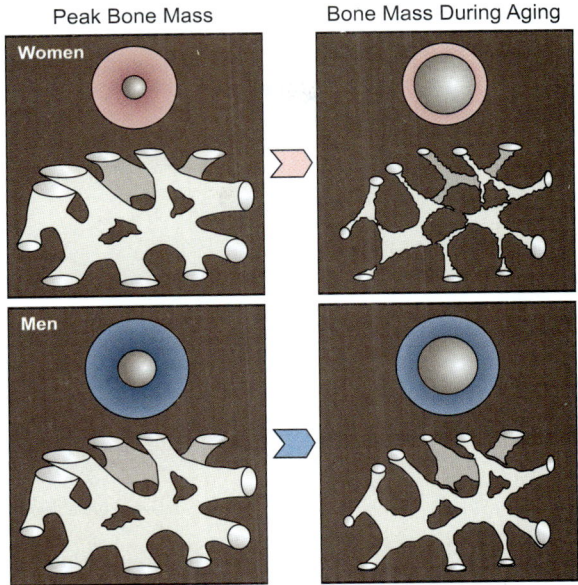

In cortical bone: Men and women lose similar amounts of cortical bone by endosteal resorption, but men have greater periosteal apposition than women, so that in men, net bone loss is less pronounced and the cortical mass is placed outward from the neutral axis, which confers them greater resistance to bending than women. *In trabecular bone*: Bone loss occurs by loss of trabecular elements in postmenopausal women and by trabecular thinning in aging men. The loss of trabecular connectivity is mainly dependent on the brisk drop of estrogen concentration due to gonadal failure and exerts a profound impact on bone strength.

Carnevale V, et al. *Arch Biochem Biophys*. 2010;503(1):110-117.

FIGURE 3.2 — The Genesis of Hip Fractures in Older Women

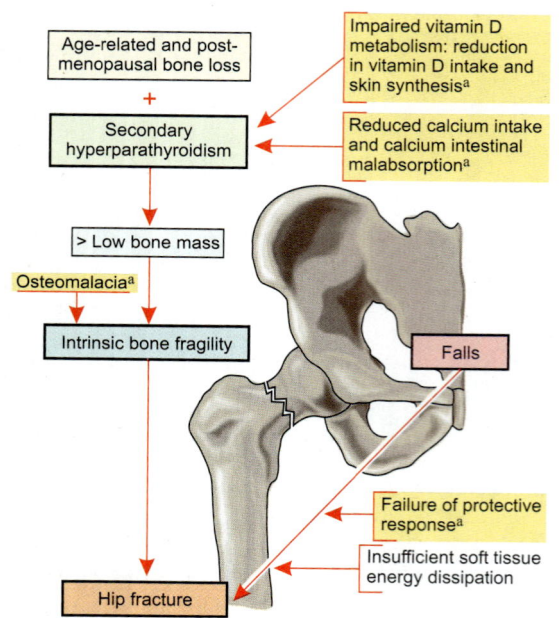

[a] Treatable/reversible factors.

promote optimal bone health in the late teens and early 20s, when bone accrual is the most rapid, are critical to prevent fractures in the aged:

- *Genetics*: The largest unmodifiable variable that determines the peak bone mass is genetics. In fact, at least 50% to 70% of genetic variance determines bone mineral density.
- *Sedentary lifestyle*: The lack of physical activity during childhood is a significant contributor to impaired peak bone mass.
- *Calcium and vitamin D deficiency*: In children and adolescents, vitamin D deficiency due to the lack of adequate sunlight parallels a sedentary

lifestyle. In fact, the incidence of rickets is increasing, especially in areas of higher latitudes where sun intensity is less.

■ Accelerated Bone Loss

Increased bone resorption that is not equally matched with the same amount of bone formation results in net bone loss. The most common causes of enhanced osteoclastic bone resorption are:

- *Estrogen deficiency*: Peri- and postmenopausal decline in estrogen accelerates bone loss in women. Estrogen reduces osteoblast RANKL and increases OPG expression and has the collective result of suppressing osteoclastogenesis.[12,13] Independent of the RANK/OPG system, estrogen can also directly promote osteoclast apoptosis.[14]

- *Calcium and vitamin D deficiency*: The lack of adequate calcium intake and vitamin D deficiency often results in secondary hyperparathyroidism. PTH production is under tight regulatory control. As serum calcium declines, as a consequence of either reduced intake or impaired intestinal absorption, the production of PTH by the parathyroid glands increases in order to restore serum calcium.[15,16] PTH operates by 1) promoting osteoblast and osteocyte production of RANKL to increase osteoclastogenesis and release bone calcium into the circulation, 2) enhancing renal calcium reabsorption, and 3) directing the renal conversion of the pro-vitamin D $25(OH)D_3$ to active $1,25(OH)_2D_3$.[17-19] Therefore, adequate dietary calcium and vitamin D are critical to prevent PTH-mediated increases in bone resorption. Age-related secondary hyperparathyroidism is preventable or reversible with vitamin D and calcium supplements. A strategy to identifying women at particular risk is to measure serum $25(OH)D_3$, with the optimal serum concentration of at least 30 ng/mL.

- *Glucocorticoids*: Osteoporosis is a nearly universal complication of long-term glucocorticoid use in patients being treated for autoimmune and chronic inflammatory diseases. Doses as little as 5 mg of oral prednisone daily promote osteoclast survival and bone resorption.[20] Even inhaled glucocorticoids may impact bone health, as measured by increased bone turnover and diminished bone mineral density.[21] Cushing's disease and primary adrenocortical overactivity also have similar effects as exogenously administered glucocorticoids.
- *Inflammatory cytokines*: Factors including IL-1, IL-6 and TNF-α directly promote osteoclast formation and survival and also increase osteoblast and inflammatory T-cell RANKL expression.[22] Inflammatory diseases such as rheumatoid arthritis and systemic lupus erythematosus, independent of glucocorticoid use, increase the risk for low bone mass and fracture.

■ Inadequate Bone Formation

The contribution of impaired bone formation to osteoporosis is less than enhanced bone resorption, but nonetheless an important factor in the pathogenesis of osteoporosis.

- *Sex steroid deficiency*: Estrogen and testosterone deficiency has the greatest effects on osteoclastic bone resorption, but recognized effects on osteoblast-dependent bone formation occur as well. Estrogen prevents osteoblast apoptosis and increases the production of IGF-1 and procollagen.[23,24]
- *Reduced growth factors*: IGF-1 has direct effects on osteoblasts to increase differentiation and bone formation.[25] Growth hormone also has positive effects on osteoblasts that are independent of IGF-1 effects.[26] GH and IGF-1 both decline with age and are correlated with declines in BMD.

- *Sedentary lifestyle*: Lack of exercise is a risk factor for fracture. This is partially due to diminished stimulation of osteocytes, the mechanical sensors in bone. Stimulation of primary cilia by fluid flow through canaliculi contributes to osteocyte sensing of bone mechanical loading.[27,28] Osteocytes respond to mechanical signals by decreasing the production of sclerostin, a secreted inhibitor of osteoblast canonical Wnt signaling, resulting in greater osteoblast differentiation.[29]
- *Glucocorticoids*: The effects of chronic glucocorticoid treatment and excess are decreased osteoblast differentiation and increased osteoblast and osteocyte apoptosis.[30] In combination with heightened osteoclastogenesis, excess glucocorticoid produces rapid declines in bone mass.

■ Poor Bone Quality

DXA is a useful tool to predict fracture risk and to monitor the effects of osteoporosis treatment (see *Chapter 5*). However, age alone is an even better predictor of fracture risk than DXA assessment and suggests that radiographic bone mineral density is only one component that predicts bone strength. "Bone quality" is the strength determined by the chemical and ultra-structural makeup of bone not measured by DXA[31]:

- *Microfractures*: Defects and small cracks in bone can initiate larger fractures.
- *Collagen arrangement*: The manner in which osteoblasts deposit collagen fibrils in forming the bone matrix determines bone strength. For example, lamellar bone is composed of collagen fibrils arranged in parallel fashion and represents mature and structurally sound bone. Woven bone is composed of disorganized collagen fibers with poor strength. This type of bone forms in situations of rapid bone formation

such as fracture repair, Paget's disease, and the osteosclerotic response to bone metastasis.

• *Degree of collagen crosslinking*: Tropocollagen is secreted by osteoblasts. Once outside the cell, enzymatic processing of these molecules cross-links large numbers of tropocollagen molecules to form a collagen fibril. The degree of collagen crosslinking determines collagen strength and ultimately bone strength.

• *Mineral to matrix ratio*: The bone matrix, composed of collagen fibrils and non-collagenous proteins, is primed for precipitation and deposition of hydroxyapatite crystals. The degree of mineral deposition is directly related to bone strength. Disorders of bone mineralization, such as rickets and osteomalacia, have defective bone matrix mineralization and poor bone strength.

Tools to measure bone quality are mostly investigational and not yet widely available for clinical practice.

■ Increased Fall Risk

Most fractures are associated with mild-to-moderate trauma superimposed on low bone mass. This is particularly true for nonvertebral fractures and is probably determined by the degree of underlying microarchitectural damage. Persons who are especially vulnerable are those with a history of previous fracture. Women with two or more previous fractures have a 6.8 to 9.0 times greater risk of future fracture compared with women with no previous fractures.

The elderly are more liable to fall because of:

• *Reduced muscle mass and strength,*[32] resulting in:
  – Slow gait with a tendency to fall backward instead of forward (**Figure 3.3**)
  – Weak leg and arm muscle strength that is responsible for the slow gait and the decreased ability to break the impact of the fall on the hip (**Figure 3.3**)

- *Reduced soft tissue*; soft tissue (fat) absorbs much of the energy generated by a fall.
- *Vitamin D deficiency* has been associated with increased fall risk.[33] Vitamin D has important direct actions on muscle function.[34,35] Replacement with cholecalciferol 700-900 IU is safe and reduces falls in the elderly. However, replacement with intermittent large doses of vitamin D (60,000-500,000 IU) may in fact increase fall risk in the elderly.[36,37] The mechanism of increased falls with very high doses is unclear.
- *Central nervous system (CNS) disorders*[38,39] causing:
    - Slowing of reflexes
    - Loss of equilibrium (vertigo and dizziness)
    - Impaired proprioception
    - Impaired vision and hearing
    - Impaired coordination
- *Drug therapy*[40] such as:
    - Hypnotics and sedatives
    - Psychotropics
    - Alcohol

Falls may be avoided when household hazards are eliminated. Steps that may be taken in the household to prevent falls include[41]:

- Exercise
- Nonslip floor surfaces
- Good illumination
- Hand rails in the bathroom
- Beds and chairs easy to get into and out of
- Fewer obstacles.

FIGURE 3.3 — Speed of Walking and the Direction of Falls

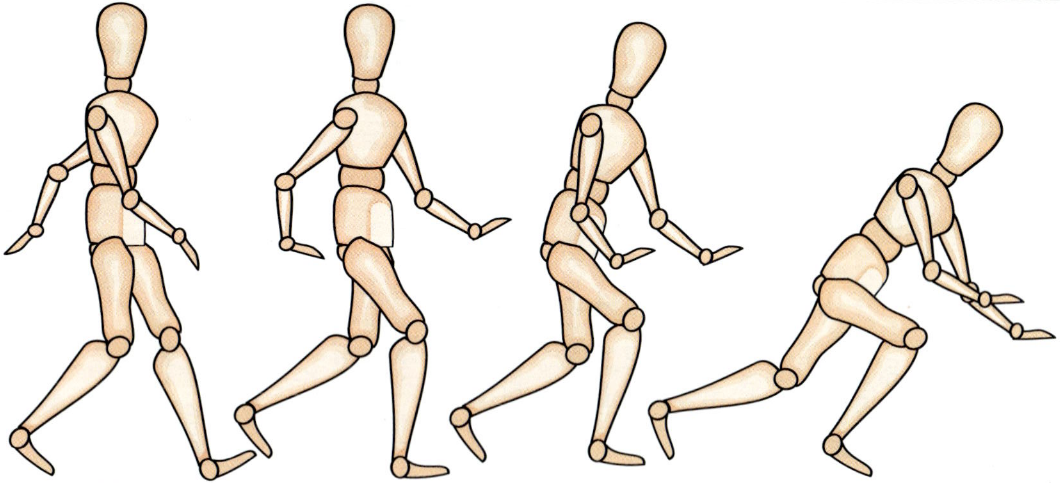

With adequate muscle strength and coordination, an individual's walking speed will result in forward falling, which will allow for protection by extension of the arms to break the fall.

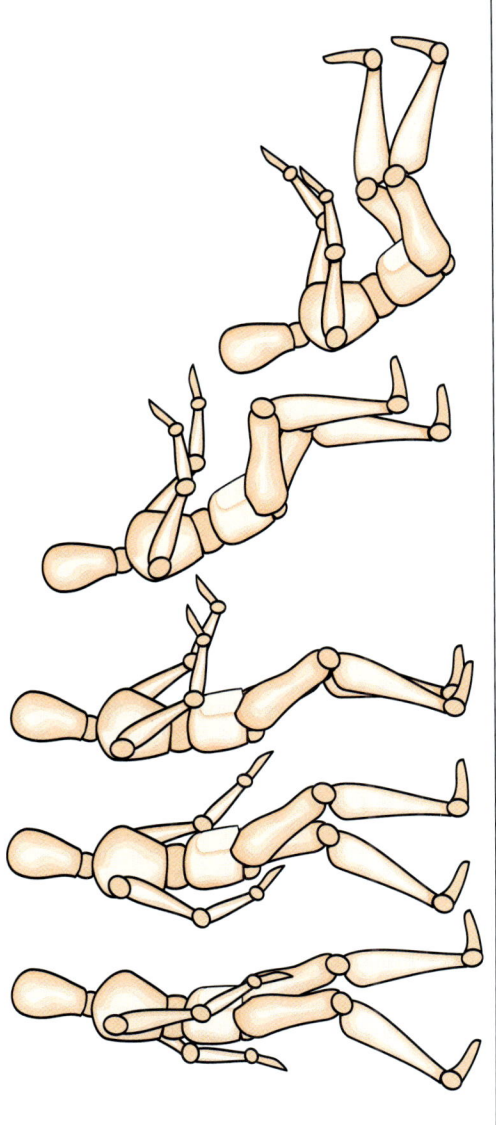

With loss of muscle strength and coordination, an individual's walking speed slows, resulting in backward falling directly onto the hip and reducing the ability to provide protection from the fall by extending the arms.

REFERENCES

1. Cummings SR, Melton LJ. Epidemiology and outcomes of osteoporotic fractures. *Lancet*. 2002;359:1761-1767.

2. Garnero P, Sornay-Rendu E, Chapuy MC, Delmas PD. Increased bone turnover in late postmenopausal women is a major determinant of osteoporosis. *J Bone Miner Res*. 1996;11: 337-349.

3. Klotzbuecher CM, Ross PD, Landsman PB, Abbott TA 3rd, Berger M. Patients with prior fractures have an increased risk of future fractures: a summary of the literature and statistical synthesis. *J Bone Miner Res*. 2000;15(4):721-739.

4. Clowes JA, Eghbali-Fatourechi GZ, McCready L, Oursler MJ, Khosla S, Riggs BL. Estrogen action on bone marrow osteoclast lineage cells of postmenopausal women in vivo. *Osteoporos Int*. 2009;20:761-769.

5. Drake MT, Khosla S. Male osteoporosis. *Endocrinol Metab Clin North Am*. 2012;41:629-641.

6. Gallet M, Saidi S, Haÿ E, et al. Repression of osteoblast maturation by ERRα accounts for bone loss induced by estrogen deficiency. *PLoS One*. 2013;8(1):e54837.

7. Farr JN, Khosla S, Miyabara Y, Miller VM, Kearns AE. Effects of estrogen with micronized progesterone on cortical and trabecular bone mass and microstructure in recently postmenopausal women. *J Clin Endocrinol Metab*. 2013;98:E249-E257.

8. Bjornerem A, Ghasem-Zadeh A, Bui M, et al. Remodeling markers are associated with larger intracortical surface area but smaller trabecular surface area: a twin study. *Bone*. 2011;49:1125-1130.

9. Heaney RP, Abrams S, Dawson-Hughes B, et al. Peak bone mass. *Osteoporos Int*. 2000;11:985-1009.

10. Baxter-Jones AD, Faulkner RA, Forwood MR, Mirwald RL, Bailey DA. Bone mineral accrual from 8 to 30 years of age: an estimation of peak bone mass. *J Bone Miner Res*. 2011;26: 1729-1739.

11. Chevalley T, Bonjour JP, van Rietbergen B, Rizzoli R, Ferrari S. Fractures in healthy females followed from childhood to early adulthood are associated with later menarcheal age and with impaired bone microstructure at peak bone mass. *J Clin Endocrinol Metab*. 2012;97:4174-4181.

12. Eghbali-Fatourechi G, Khosla S, Sanyal A, Boyle WJ, Lacey DL, Riggs BL. Role of RANK ligand in mediating increased bone resorption in early postmenopausal women. *J Clin Invest*. 2003;111:1221-1230.

13. Hofbauer LC, Khosla S, Dunstan CR, Lacey DL, Spelsberg TC, Riggs BL. Estrogen stimulates gene expression and protein production of osteoprotegerin in human osteoblastic cells. *Endocrinology*. 1999;140:4367-4370.

14. Hughes DE, Dai A, Tiffee JC, Li HH, Mundy GR, Boyce BF. Estrogen promotes apoptosis of murine osteoclasts mediated by TGF-beta. *Nat Med*. 1996;2:1132-1136.

15. Brown EM, Gamba G, Riccardi D, et al. Cloning and characterization of an extracellular $Ca(2+)$-sensing receptor from bovine parathyroid. *Nature*. 1993;366:575-580.

16. Brown EM, MacLeod RJ. Extracellular calcium sensing and extracellular calcium signaling. *Physiol Rev*. 2001;81:239-297.

17. van Abel M, Hoenderop JG, van der Kemp AW, Friedlaender MM, van Leeuwen JP, Bindels RJ. Coordinated control of renal $Ca(2+)$ transport proteins by parathyroid hormone. *Kidney Int*. 2005;68:1708-1721.

18. Xiong J, Onal M, Jilka RL, Weinstein RS, Manolagas SC, O'Brien CA. Matrix-embedded cells control osteoclast formation. *Nat Med*. 2011;17:1235-1241.

19. Huang JC, Sakata T, Pfleger LL, et al. PTH differentially regulates expression of RANKL and OPG. *J Bone Miner Res*. 2004;19:235-244.

20. van Staa TP, Leufkens HG, Abenhaim L, Zhang B, Cooper C. Oral corticosteroids and fracture risk: relationship to daily and cumulative doses. *Rheumatology (Oxford)*. 2000;39:1383-1389.

21. Emkey RD, Lindsay R, Lyssy J, Weisberg JS, Dempster DW, Shen V. The systemic effect of intraarticular administration of corticosteroid on markers of bone formation and bone resorption in patients with rheumatoid arthritis. *Arthritis Rheum*. 1996;39:277-282.

22. Walsh NC, Crotti TN, Goldring SR, Gravallese EM. Rheumatic diseases: the effects of inflammation on bone. *Immunol Rev*. 2005;208:228-251.

23. Chow J, Tobias JH, Colston KW, Chambers TJ. Estrogen maintains trabecular bone volume in rats not only by suppression of bone resorption but also by stimulation of bone formation. *J Clin Invest*. 1992;89:74-78.

3

24. Ernst M, Heath JK, Rodan GA. Estradiol effects on proliferation, messenger ribonucleic acid for collagen and insulin-like growth factor-I, and parathyroid hormone-stimulated adenylate cyclase activity in osteoblastic cells from calvariae and long bones. *Endocrinology.* 1989;125:825-833.

25. Bikle D, Majumdar S, Laib A, et al. The skeletal structure of insulin-like growth factor I-deficient mice. *J Bone Miner Res.* 2001;16:2320-2329.

26. DiGirolamo DJ, Mukherjee A, Fulzele K, et al. Mode of growth hormone action in osteoblasts. *J Biol Chem.* 2007;282:31666-31674.

27. Turner CH, Forwood MR, Otter MW. Mechanotransduction in bone: do bone cells act as sensors of fluid flow? *FASEB J.* 1994;8:875-878.

28. Malone AM, Anderson CT, Tummala P, et al. Primary cilia mediate mechanosensing in bone cells by a calcium-independent mechanism. *Proc Natl Acad Sci USA.* 2007;104:13325-13330.

29. Robling AG, Niziolek PJ, Baldridge LA, et al. Mechanical stimulation of bone in vivo reduces osteocyte expression of Sost/sclerostin. *J Biol Chem.* 2008;283:5866-5875.

30. O'Brien CA, Jia D, Plotkin LI, et al. Glucocorticoids act directly on osteoblasts and osteocytes to induce their apoptosis and reduce bone formation and strength. *Endocrinology.* 2004;145:1835-1841.

31. Seeman E, Delmas PD. Bone quality--the material and structural basis of bone strength and fragility. *N Engl J Med.* 2006;354:2250-2261.

32. Skelton DA. Effects of physical activity on postural stability. *Age Ageing.* 2001;30(suppl 4):33-39.

33. Bischoff-Ferrari HA, Dawson-Hughes B, Willett WC, et al. Effect of Vitamin D on falls: a meta-analysis. *JAMA.* 2004;291:1999-2006.

34. Girgis CM, Clifton-Bligh RJ, Hamrick MW, Holick MF, Gunton JE. The roles of vitamin d in skeletal muscle: form, function, and metabolism. *Endocr Rev.* 2013;34:33-83.

35. Bischoff-Ferrari HA, Dawson-Hughes B, Staehelin HB, et al. Fall prevention with supplemental and active forms of vitamin D: a meta-analysis of randomised controlled trials. *BMJ.* 2009;339:b3692.

36. Sanders KM, Stuart AL, Williamson EJ, et al. Annual high-dose oral vitamin D and falls and fractures in older women: a randomized controlled trial. *JAMA.* 2010;303(18):1815-1822.

37. Bischoff-Ferrari HA, Dawson-Hughes B, Orav EJ, et al. Monthly high-dose vitamin D treatment for the prevention of functional decline: a randomized clinical trial. *JAMA Intern Med.* 2016;176(2):175-183.

38. van Doorn C, Gruber-Baldini AL, Zimmerman S, et al. Dementia as a risk factor for falls and fall injuries among nursing home residents. *J Am Geriatr Soc.* 2003;51:1213-1218.

39. Krauss MJ, Evanoff B, Hitcho E, et al. A case-control study of patient, medication, and care-related risk factors for inpatient falls. *J Gen Intern Med.* 2005;20:116-122.

40. Woolcott JC, Richardson KJ, Wiens MO, et al. Meta-analysis of the impact of 9 medication classes on falls in elderly persons. *Arch Intern Med.* 2009;169:1952-1960.

41. Oliver D, Connelly JB, Victor CR, et al. Strategies to prevent falls and fractures in hospitals and care homes and effect of cognitive impairment: systematic review and meta-analyses. *BMJ.* 2007;334:82.

3

4

Diagnosis: History, Risk Factors, and Physical Examination

Clinical assessment of patients with suspected osteoporosis should include a detailed history and a focused clinical examination. In addition to evaluation of the musculoskeletal system, a general examination should be performed to look for underlying diseases that are associated with osteoporosis.

Evaluation of the Patient— Taking an Osteoporosis History

Identifying the patient at risk for osteoporosis is an important and often challenging responsibility. Women traditionally considered most at risk are white or Asian, with a family history of osteoporosis, a petite, small frame, a previous insufficiency fracture before the age of 40 or long-term use of oral glucocorticoids. Historical risk factors are poor predictors of bone mineral density (BMD), but can be useful in the prediction of future fracture risk. Risk factors for bone loss are shown in **Table 4.1**.

In patients with suspected osteoporosis, risk factors should be documented, including:
- Previous fractures, suspicious height loss, or back pain
- Fall history
- Use of medications known to affect bone mass
- Intake of calcium and vitamin D via diet, sunlight, and supplements
- Family history of osteoporosis and/or hip fracture.

These risk factors are described in more detail below.

TABLE 4.1 — Conditions, Diseases, and Medications That Cause or Contribute to Osteoporosis and Fractures

Lifestyle Factors
Alcohol abuse
Low calcium intake
Vitamin D insufficiency
Excess vitamin A
High salt intake
Inadequate physical activity
Immobilization
Smoking (active or passive)
Frequent falling
Excessive thinness

Genetic Factors
Cystic fibrosis
Ehlers-Danlos
Gaucher's disease
Glycogen storage diseases
Hemochromatosis
Homocystinuria
Hypophosphatasia
Marfan syndrome
Menkes steely hair syndrome
Osteogenesis imperfecta
Parental history of hip fracture
Porphyria
Riley-Day syndrome

Hypogonadal States
Androgen insensitivity
Anorexia nervosa
Turner's and Klinefelter's syndromes
Hyperprolactinemia
Premature menopause (<40 y)
Athletic amenorrhea
Panhypopituitarism

Endocrine Disorders

Diabetes mellitus (types 1 and 2) Cushing's syndrome Central obesity
Hyperparathyroidism Thyrotoxicosis

Gastrointestinal Disorders

Celiac disease Inflammatory bowel disease Primary biliary cirrhosis
Gastric bypass Malabsorption
Gastrointestinal surgery

Hematologic Disorders

Multiple myeloma Monoclonal gammopathies Sickle cell disease
Hemophilia Leukemia and lymphomas Systemic mastocytosis
Thalassemia

Rheumatologic and Autoimmune Diseases

Ankylosing spondylitis Systemic lupus Rheumatoid arthritis
Other rheumatic and autoimmune diseases

Neurological and Musculoskeletal Risk Factors

Epilepsy Parkinson's disease Stroke
Multiple sclerosis Spinal cord injury Muscular dystrophy

Continued

4

TABLE 4.1 — Continued

Miscellaneous Conditions and Diseases

AIDS/HIV	Congestive heart failure	Post-transplant bone disease
Amyloidosis	Depression	Sarcoidosis
Chronic metabolic acidosis	End-stage renal disease	Weight loss
Chronic obstructive lung disease	Hypercalciuria	Idiopathic scoliosis

Medications

Aluminum (in antacids)	Depo-medroxyprogesterone (premenopausal contraception)	Proton pump inhibitors
Anticoagulants (heparin)		Selective serotonin reuptake inhibitors
Anticonvulsants	Glucocorticoids (≥5 mg/day prednisone or equivalent for ≥3 mo)	Tamoxifen (premenopausal use)
Aromatase inhibitors		Thiazolidinediones (such as pioglitazone and rosiglitazone)
Barbiturates	GnRH (gonadotropin-releasing hormone) agonists	Thyroid hormones (in excess)
Cancer chemotherapeutic drugs	Lithium cyclosporin A and tacrolimus	Parental nutrition
Methotrexate		

Adapted from Cosman F, et al. *Osteoporos Int.* 2014;25:2359-2381.

Non-modifiable Risk Factors

■ **Genetics**

Peak bone mass is the maximum BMD reached during a lifetime, usually by approximately age 20.[1,2] In addition to bone loss associated with aging, low bone mass in adults may be due to low peak bone mass in early adulthood—which is a risk factor for osteoporosis. Approximately 60% to 80% of peak bone mass is dependent on genetics. Moreover, certain genetic diseases, such as osteogenesis imperfecta and hemochromatosis and parental history of hip fracture, are risk factors for osteoporosis.

Modifiable Risk Factors

■ **Lifestyle Risk Factors**

Risk factors that are modifiable and may accelerate bone loss include:

- A diet deficient in vitamin D and calcium. An assessment of dietary calcium intake should be conducted; methods utilizing tables that list calcium-containing foods and their calcium content are readily available, and can be calculated by the patient (see *Chapter 8*). Calcium supplements are used by many patients. Patients should also be asked about their exposure to sunlight and dietary and supplemental vitamin D intake.
- Inactivity or immobilization
- Excessive intake of alcohol
- Smoking
- Low BMI

Gynecologic Risk Factors

Women are especially at risk if they have had a premature or early surgical menopause and have not received hormone therapy (HT) after menopause.[3,4]

■ **Late Menarche**

The onset of the menarche is an important biologic indicator of future bone mass; the earlier the onset of menstruation, the greater the individual's subsequent bone mass. With closure of the epiphysis, longitudinal bone growth ceases, but endosteal bone apposition continues for a variable period of time. Areal BMD in both cortical and trabecular bone increases markedly during puberty. Given the dynamic activity of the bone-remodeling cycle during puberty, this is an important time to influence bone mass accrual with interventions such as exercise and optimal nutrition.

■ **Menstrual History**

Disturbance of the menstrual cycle may affect bone health. Late menarche and irregular menstrual cycles and early menopause are associated with reduced bone mass. In one study, women with an early menopause had a 15% lower BMD than women who had menopause that occurred later.[3,4] Early menopause before the age of 51 years is also associated with osteoporotic fractures before the age of 70. Women with the female athletic triad (the effect of energy availability on BMD and menstrual function) often have low peak BMD[5] (see anorexia nervosa below).

■ **Pregnancy and Lactation**

Increased number of births does not appear to increase the risk of osteoporosis. In a study of post-menopausal women who had given birth ≥10 times compared with matched women who had given birth ≤3 times, there was no difference in spine or hip bone mineral density.[6] Increased calcium needs during pregnancy are met by increased calcium absorption and increased synthesis of $1,25\,(OH)_2$ vitamin D with a relative absorptive hypercalciuria.[7]

Extended lactation is associated with physiologic bone loss. However, BMD may improve and generally returns to baseline levels within a year after a woman gives birth.[8] It is generally felt that long-term breast feeding is not a risk factor for later lower BMD and women who have breastfed >33 months in their life had greater bone strength and bone size compared with women who had breastfed <12 months in their life.[9-11] However, adolescent pregnancy at a time that peak bone mass is being accrued has been found to be associated with an increased fracture risk in postmenopausal women.[12] Multiparity and prolonged lactation have been found to have a negative impact on BMD in groups of women with borderline nutritional intake.[13]

■ **Hysterectomy**

Premenopausal women who have had a hysterectomy with retention of their ovaries have bone density that is significantly lower than normal menstruating controls.[14] It is not known whether this bone loss is due to aberrant functioning of the retained ovaries.

■ **Menopausal Status**

Owing to changes in perimenopausal estrogen production, bone loss accelerates within to 2 to 3 years before the cessation of menstruation, ending 3 to 4 years after menopause.[15-18] Perimenopausal bone loss is about 2% annually and slows to approximately 1% to 1.5% per year thereafter. There is particularly a loss of trabecular BMD in the spine during the first 5 postmenopausal years. There is a strong association between these lower estrogen levels and an increased fracture risk in older women.

Eating Disorders

■ **Anorexia Nervosa**

Patients with anorexia nervosa have significantly reduced bone mass compared with normal controls.[19-25] The presence of an eating disorder is also predictive of a higher subsequent risk of fracture. Numerous factors, including estrogen deficiency, IGF-1 deficiency, GH resistance, low DHEA-S levels, hypercortisolemia, ghrelin resistance, increased osteoprotegerin, reduced leptin levels, malnutrition including low calcium and vitamin D intake, and low T_3 levels have been postulated to have a role in low bone mass in these individuals. Clinical determinants of low bone mass in anorexia include presentation at a younger age before menarche, duration of the anorexia, duration of amenorrhea, estrogen deprivation exposure time, low body mass index, subtype of anorexia with the binge-eating purging type being more at risk than the restrictive type, frequency of vomiting, and depression. While, bone mass often improves with a cure of the eating disorder, not all individuals cured from anorexia nervosa will have a rebound in BMD. However, one follow-up study of anorectic individuals found that 2 years of treatment with calcium, exercise, and estrogen resulted in most patients gaining weight but, unfortunately, no improvement in bone mass. In anorexia nervosa, the data are conflicting about the usefulness of hormones to improve BMD.[25,26] While high-dose estrogen has been shown not to improve BMD,[25] physiologic estradiol doses that mimic puberty have been found to increase BMD.[26]

■ The Female Athletic Triad

The female athletic triad includes disordered eating, amenorrhea, and low bone mass. It is important to closely monitor the thin oligomenorrheic or amenorrheic athlete.[5,19] Additional information from the Female Athlete Triad Coalition is available at www.femaleathletetriad.org.[19]

Endocrinopathies as Risk Factors

Table 4.1 lists endocrine disorders that cause osteoporosis.[27] Osteoporosis occurs in patients with hypoestrogenism due to gonadal dysgenesis (Turner's syndrome) and premature ovarian failure, irrespective of the cause. A less obvious cause of low bone mass is hyperprolactinemia.[28,29] The pathogenesis of bone loss associated with hyperprolactinemia is incompletely understood and hyperprolactinemia may be seen with use of antipsychotic medications. Hyperthyroidism, and over-replacement with thyroid hormone, are also risk factors for bone loss.

Gastrointestinal Diseases as Risk Factors

Table 4.1 lists some gastrointestinal diseases associated with low bone mass. Gastrointestinal diseases may be a risk factor for osteoporosis through a variety of mechanisms including malabsorption of calcium and vitamin D and maldigestion/malabsorption of other nutrients, problems with the formation of 25-OH vitamin D (advanced liver disease), acidosis, the inflammatory state, and the use of medications such as glucocorticoids.[30-34] Celiac disease is an example of a gastrointestinal disorder that untreated is associated with low bone mass and calcium and vitamin D malabsorption. Adherence to a gluten-free diet is important in this population. Patients with obesity surgeries which bypass the small bowel have also been documented to have problems with malabsorption and subsequent loss of BMD depending on the extent and location of the bypassed small bowel.

Medications as Risk Factors

Table 4.1 lists medications associated with bone loss.[15,35,36] Loss of BMD with glucocorticoid use begins within the first 3 months of use and peaks by approximately 6 months, with continued loss with chronic use. Anticonvulsants (phenytoin, carbamazepine, and valproate) affect vitamin D metabolism and are often related to loss of BMD. The effect of new anticonvulsants (topiramate, gabapentin, vigabatrin, levetiracetam, oxcarbazepine, and lamotrigine) is being studied.[37-40] Medications associated with low bone mass and fractures are discussed in *Chapter 11*.

Fall Risk Factors

Risk factors for falling should be assessed, such as use of sedatives, neurologic disease, cardiovascular disorders, and visual impairment. More than 25% of persons >65 years of age fall at least once annually; 5% of these falls will result in a fracture. Falls may be due to many factors, including neurologic or cardiovascular disease, orthostatic hypotension, and impaired musculoskeletal function. A recent analysis shows increasing fall rates in both young and older men and women.[41]

In screening for a tendency to fall, women should be asked whether they experience dizziness. Dizziness can present as vertigo, syncope, and lightheadedness. Vertigo is associated with a sense of rotation of either the patient or the environment, and is almost always associated with nystagmus, poor balance, and autonomic symptoms. Vestibular dysfunction is usually the primary problem. Syncope is defined as a brief loss of consciousness due to cerebral ischemia, vasovagal attacks, orthostatic hypotension, carotid sinus syncope, or cardiac abnormalities, all of which need to be evaluated. Dizziness without nystagmus or loss of consciousness may occur in many conditions including hypoglycemia, hypothyroidism, hyperventilation, and visual malfunction. It is also important to inquire about fall risks in the home such as loose rugs, the absence of grab bars in the shower/bathroom, inadequate handrails on stairs, and inadequate use of ambulatory assistance devices such as canes and walkers.

Visual impairment is an important risk factor for falling and fractures. Different aspects of vision are involved including visual acuity, visual field, and contrast sensitivity. The latter refers to the ability to differentiate between two objects of different light intensity. Contrast sensitivity integrates and reflects the total amount of visual information assimilated by the visual system. Women with poor visual contrast sensitivity have an increased risk of falling. Regular eye examinations are important.

FRAX as a Risk-Assessment Tool

Although measurement of BMD provides a good assessment of fracture risk (see *Chapter 5*), this can be improved by the addition of certain clinical risk factors that are to some extent independent of BMD. In 2008, FRAX®, an algorithm that incorporates clinical factors to determine fracture risk was released.[42-46] **Figure 4.1** shows a screenshot of the FRAX® tool which can be accessed at www.sheffield.ac.uk/FRAX/. FRAX® can be used with or without femoral neck BMD. The FRAX® calculator has the ability to also insert QCT data and may be modified for TBS (see *Chapter 5*). It estimates the 10-year absolute probability of hip fracture, as well as major osteoporotic fracture (hip, clinical vertebral, proximal humerus, distal forearm) in untreated men and women from the age of 40 to 90. Demographic parameters used with FRAX® include age, sex, weight, and femoral neck BMD, where available (**Table 4.2**).

FIGURE 4.1 — Fracture Risk Assessment Tool: FRAX®a

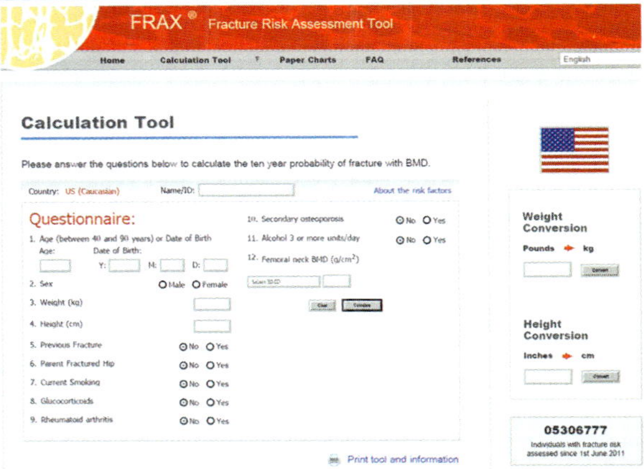

a Calculates the 10 year probability of hip and major osteoporotic fractures in previously untreated patients based on risk factor, including BMD.

FRAX® Fracture Risk Assessment Tool Web site. http://www.sheffield.ac.uk/FRAX/. Accessed May 30, 2017.

TABLE 4.2 — Risk Factors for FRAX®

- Current age
- Gender
- Prior osteoporotic fracture (including morphometric vertebral fracture)
- Femoral neck BMD
- Low body mass index (kg/m²)
- Rheumatoid arthritis
- Secondary osteoporosis
- Parental history of hip fracture
- Current smoking
- Alcohol intake (≥3 drinks/day)
- Oral glucocorticoids ≥5 mg/day of prednisone for ≥3 months (ever)

Notes on FRAX® Risk Factors

Previous Fracture

A special situation pertains to a prior history of vertebral fracture. A fracture detected as a radiographic observation alone (a morphometric vertebral fracture) counts as a previous fracture. A prior clinical vertebral fracture or a hip fracture is an especially strong risk factor. The probability of fracture computed may therefore be underestimated. Fracture probability is also underestimated with multiple fractures.

Smoking, Alcohol, Glucocorticoids

These risk factors appear to have a dose-dependent effect, ie, the higher the exposure, the greater the risk. This is not taken into account and the computations assume average exposure. Clinical judgment should be used for low or high exposures.

Rheumatoid Arthritis (RA)

RA is a risk factor for fracture. However, osteoarthritis is, if anything, protective. For this reason, reliance should not be placed on a patient's report of "arthritis" unless there is clinical or laboratory evidence to support the diagnosis.

Bone Mineral Density (BMD)

The site and reference technology is DXA at the femoral neck. T-scores are based on the NHANES reference values for women aged 20-29 years. The same absolute values are used in men.

Continued

TABLE 4.2 — *Continued*

WHO Technical Report: Kanis JA, on behalf of the World Health Organization Scientific Group. Assessment of Osteoporosis at the Primary Health Care Level. 2008 Technical Report: University of Sheffield, UK: WHO Collaborating Center; 2008; FRAX®: Fracture Risk Assessment Tool Web site. http://www.sheffield. ac.uk/FRAX/. Accessed May 31, 2017.

The development of FRAX® was based on prospective analysis of about 60,000 men and women in Europe, North America, Asia, and Australia. It was then corroborated in independent cohorts totaling more than 230,000 subjects. This tool can be customized for any country or ethnic group where specific fracture and mortality rates are available.

Although FRAX® has become a widely accepted prognostic tool for assessing fracture risk, it does not take into account certain parameters that may affect fracture probability (see *Chapter 5* for a discussion of other fracture risk calculators). FRAX:

- Does not include falls as a variable and may therefore underestimate probability in individuals with a history of falls
- Underestimates fracture probability where there is a history of multiple fractures
- May underestimate fracture probability in individuals with undiagnosed prevalent vertebral fractures
- Only femoral neck BMD, and not spine BMD, can be used. However, a correction calculation to modify the FRAX® for low spinal BMD is available.[47,48]
- Does not quantify risk of smoking or alcohol abuse based on duration and dose
- Dose and duration of glucocorticoid therapy are not accommodated
- Applies only to untreated patients, although studies have indicated that it may applied to treated patients
- Is limited to ages 40-90.[49]

Physical Examination

■ **Height, Weight, Blood Pressure**

Height and weight should be measured. Loss of height may be the patient's first sign of vertebral fracture. Height is only lost in the vertebral column; the hip-to-heel length remains constant. Serial measurements of height, (for example annually), using a stadiometer provides a more accurate means of evaluating height loss over time. A loss of height of two inches or more is associated with a significant risk for vertebral compression fractures. The body mass index (BMI) is calculated either by hand or using various nomograms found on the internet. The BMI is determined by the formula weight in kilograms/height in meters squared:

$$BMI = \frac{weight\ (kg)}{height\ (m^2)}$$

Weight is influenced by both lean and fat body mass, and a more detailed body composition assessment can be made using DXA or other methods.

Low BMI is a significant risk factor for osteoporosis. Age–related loss of strength and muscle mass is called sarcopenia and is associated with low BMD.[50] Values of BMI ≥ 30 kg/m^2 are indicative of obesity. Although it was previously believed that obesity was protective against fracture, recent studies suggest that the risk of certain fractures, particularly of the ankle and lower leg, are increased in obese postmenopausal women.[51]

Persons experiencing falls associated with dizziness should be tested for orthostatic hypotension. The blood pressure should be taken in a supine or sitting position and repeated with the patient standing. The patient's blood pressure should be measured within 30 seconds of standing and again 3 minutes later. A drop in systolic blood pressure of 20 mm Hg and 10 mm Hg in diastolic pressure is indicative of postural hypotension. If the pulse rate does not increase, a primary autonomic disturbance is the probable cause of the hypotension. A benefit of the Garvan fracture risk calculator is that falls are factored into fracture risk (see *Chapter 5*).

■ General and Musculoskeletal Examination

The general physical examination typically provides few clues as to the presence of osteoporosis or its associated risk factors. Uncommon secondary causes may be uncovered or suspected on the basis of findings on physical examination[52] (**Table 4.3**).

The patient's posture and the shape of the spine may provide valuable clinical clues. Dorsal kyphosis, scoliosis, the presence/absence of appropriate lumbar lordosis, shoulder height, leg length disparity, and pelvic tilt or rotation are all important clinical signs. Much of the back pain experienced by patients with vertebral fractures is muscular in origin. There may be localized tenderness at the site of fracture and restriction of spinal movement.

Disparity in leg length is associated with both hip and low back pain and may cause imbalance and a risk for falling. It is also associated with an increased risk of stress fractures. Measurements are usually taken from the anterior superior iliac crest to the medial malleolus (**Figure 4.2-A**). **Figures 4.2-B** and **4.2-C** also illustrate how observation of flexed knees placed side by side with the patient supine can differentiate between leg-length disparity due to the femur or lower leg.[53]

TABLE 4.3 — Physical Examination Findings of Metabolic and Genetic Bone Disorders

Physical Finding	Suggested Diagnosis
Alopecia	Hereditary vitamin D-resistant rickets (HVDRR)
Enlarged skull	Paget's disease, hypophosphatemic rickets
Dental defects	X-linked hypophosphatemic rickets, osteogenesis imperfecta
Round face	Cushing syndrome
Blue or gray sclerae	Osteogenesis imperfecta
Dorsocervial fat pad	Cushing syndrome
Gynecomastia	Hypogonadism (osteoporosis risk ractor)
Spinal tenderness	Occult vertebral compression fracture
Abdominal scars	Gastrectomy, other GI surgery that can lead to malabsorption
Proximal muscle wasting and weakness	Osteomalacia, Cushing syndrome
Small testes and/or soft testes	Hypogonadism (osteoporosis risk factor)
Anterior tibial tenderness	Osteomalacia
Deformed bones	Paget's disease, rickets, renal osteodystrophy
Redness and warmth over a bone	Paget's disease
Joint laxity	Osteogenesis imperfecta
Arthritic changes in joints	Rheumatoid arthritis, inflammatory bowel disease
Vascular calcifications	Renal osteodystrophy

REFERENCES

1. Weaver CM, Gordon CM, Janz KF, et al. The National Osteoporosis Foundation's position statement on peak bone mass development and lifestyle factors: a systematic review and implementation recommendations. *Osteoporos Int.* 2016;27:1281-1386.

2. Gordon CM, Zemel BS, Wren TA, et al. The determinants of peak bone mass. *J Pediatr.* 2017;180:261-269.

3. Gallagher JC. Effect of early menopause on bone mineral density and fractures. *Menopause.* 2007;14(3 Pt 2):567-571.

4. Pouilles JM, Tremollieres F, Bonneu M, et al. Influence of early age at menopause on vertebral bone mass. *J Bone Miner Res.* 1994;9(3):311-315.

5. Nissenbaum-Thein J, Hammer E. Treatment strategies for the female athlete triad in the adolescent athlete: current perspectives. *Open Access J Sports Med.* 2017;8:85-95.

6. Turan V. Grand-grand multiparity (more than 10 deliveries) does not convey a risk for osteoporosis. *Acta Obstet Gynecol Scand.* 2011;90(12):1440-1442.

7. Mahadevan S, Kumaravel V, Bharath R. Calcium and bone disorders in pregnancy. *Indian J Endocrinol Metab.* 2012;16:358-363.

8. Sowers FM, Corton G, Shaprio B, et al. Changes in bone density with lactation. *JAMA.* 1993;269:3130-3135.

9. Kovacs CS. Calcium and bone metabolism disorders during pregnancy and lactation. *Endocrinol Metab Clin North Am.* 2011;40(4):795-826.

10. Wiklund PK, Xu L, Wang Q, et al. Lactation is associated with greater maternal bone size and bone strength later in life. *Osteoporos Int.* 2012;23(7):1939-1945.

11. Yazici S, Korkmaz U, Erkan M, et al. The effect of breast-feeding duration on bone mineral density in postmenopausal Turkish women: a population-based study. *Arch Med Sci.* 2011;7(3):486-492.

12. Cho GJ, Shin JH, Yi KW, et al. Adolescent pregnancy is associated with osteoporosis in postmenopausal women. *Menopause.* 2012;19:456-460, 2012.

13. Sharma N, Natung T, Rituparna B, and Ahanthem SS. Effect of multiparity and prolonged lactation on bone mineral density. *J Menopausal Med.* 2016;22:161-166.

FIGURE 4.2 — Assessing Leg-Length Discrepancies

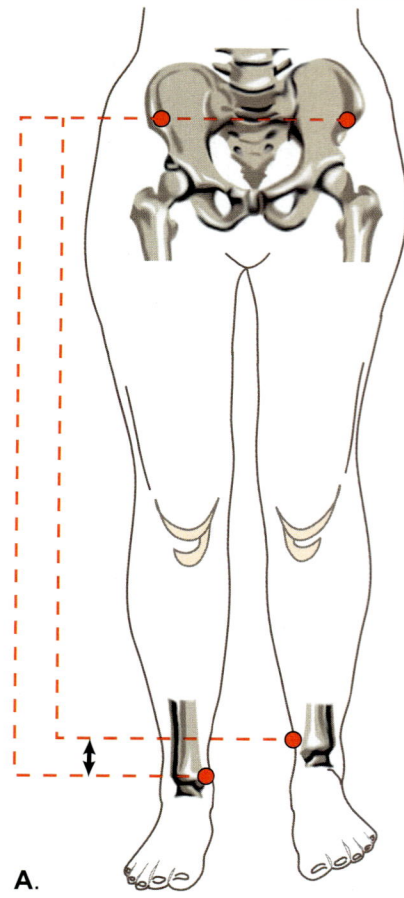

A.

Continued

FIGURE 4.2 — *Continued*

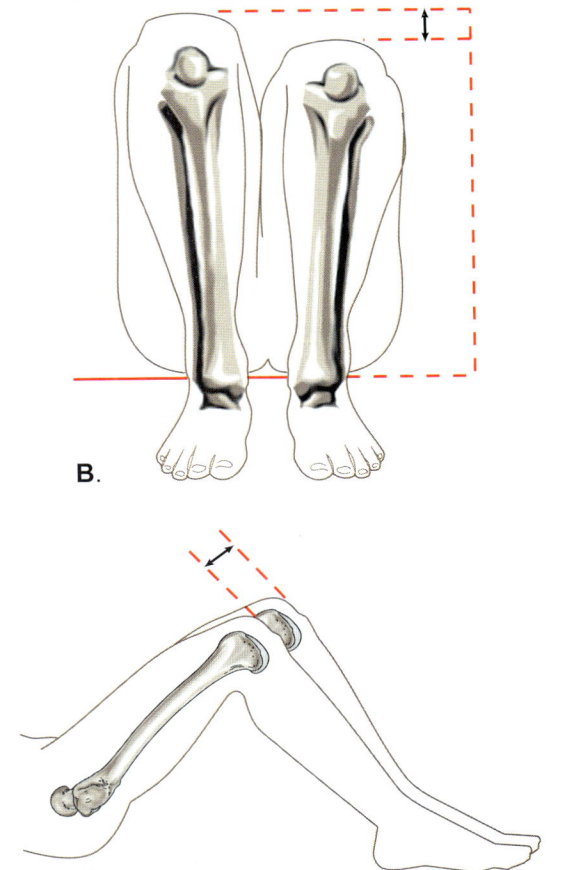

B.

C.

14. Cheng S, Sievanen H, Heinonen A, et al. Does hysterectomy with ovarian conservation affect bone metabolism and density? *J Bone Miner Metab.* 2003;21(1):12-16.

15. Rizzoli R, Adachi JD, Cooper C, et al. Management of glucocorticoid-induced osteoporosis. *Calcif Tissue Int.* 2012; 91(4):225-243.

16. Rosen CJ. Clinical practice. Postmenopausal osteoporosis. *N Engl J Med.* 2005;353(6):595-603.

17. Schnatz PF, Marakovits KA, O'Sullivan DM. Assessment of postmenopausal women and significant risk factors for osteoporosis. *Obstet Gynecol Surv.* 2010;65(9):591-596.

18. Watts NB, Bilezikian JP, Camacho PM, et al. American Association of Clinical Endocrinologists Medical Guidelines for Clinical Practice for the diagnosis and treatment of postmenopausal osteoporosis. *Endocr Pract.* 2010;16(suppl 3):1-37.

19. Female Athlete Triad Coalition: An International Consortium.

20. Jayasinghe Y, Grover SR, Zacharin M. Current concepts in bone and reproductive health in adolescents with anorexia nervosa. *BJOG.* 2008;115(3):304-315.

21. Jonnavithula S, Warren MP, Fox RP, et al. Bone density is compromised in amenorrheic women despite return of menses: a 2-year study. *Obstet Gynecol.* 1993;81(5 Pt 1):669-674.

22. Lucas AR, Melton LJ 3rd, Crowson CS, et al. Long-term fracture risk among women with anorexia nervosa: a population-based cohort study. *Mayo Clin Proc.* 1999;74(10):972-927.

23. Mehler PS, MacKenzie TD. Treatment of osteopenia and osteoporosis in anorexia nervosa: a systematic review of the literature. *Int J Eat Disord.* 2009;42(3):195-201.

24. Mendelsohn FA, Warren MP. Anorexia, bulimia, and the female athlete triad: evaluation and management. *Endocrinol Metab Clin North Am.* 2010;39(1):155-167, x.

25. Sim LA, McGovern L, Elamin MB, et al. Effect on bone health of estrogen preparations in premenopausal women with anorexia nervosa: a systematic review and meta-analyses. *Int J Eat Disord.* 2010;43(3):218-225.

26. Misra M, Katzman D, Miller KK, et al. Physiologic estrogen replacement increases bone density in adolescent girls with anorexia nervosa. *J Bone Miner Res.* 2011;26:2340-2438.

27. Dutta D, Dharmshaktu P, Aggarwal A, et al. Severity and pattern of bone mineral loss in endocrine causes of osteoporosis as compared to age-related bone mineral loss. *J Postgrad Med.* 2016;62:162-169.

28. Inder WJ, Castle D. Antipsychotic-induced hyperprolactinae-mia. *Aust N Z J Psychiatry*. 2011;45(10):830-837.

29. Shibli-Rahhal A, Schlechte J. The effects of hyperprolactinemia on bone and fat. *Pituitary*. 2009;12(2):96-104.

30. Casella S, Zanini B, Lanzarotto F, et al. Celiac disease in elderly adults: clinical, serological, and histological charac-teristics and the effect of a gluten-free diet. *J Am Geriatr Soc*. 2012;60(6):1064-1069.

31. Duggan SN, O'Sullivan M, Hamilton S, et al. Patients with chronic pancreatitis are at increased risk for osteoporosis. *Pancreas*. 2012;41(7):1119-1124.

32. Etzel JP, Larson MF, Anawalt BD, et al. Assessment and man-agement of low bone density in inflammatory bowel disease and performance of professional society guidelines. *Inflamm Bowel Dis*. 2011;17(10):2122-2129.

33. Khan MA, Morgan SL. Tone the bones of your chronic liver disease patients. *Clin Gastroenterol Hepatol*. 2009;7(8):814-815.

34. Mechanick JI, Kushner RF, Sugerman HJ, et al. American Association of Clinical Endocrinologists, The Obesity Society, and American Society for Metabolic & Bariatric Surgery Medical guidelines for clinical practice for the perioperative nutritional, metabolic, and nonsurgical support of the bariatric surgery patient. *Endocr Pract*. 2008;14(suppl 1):1-83.

35. Grossman JM, Gordon R, Ranganath VK, et al. American College of Rheumatology 2010 recommendations for the pre-vention and treatment of glucocorticoid-induced osteoporosis. *Arthritis Care Res (Hoboken)*. 2010;62(11):1515-1526.

36. Lee RH, Lyles KW, Sloane R, Colón-Emeric C. The association of newer anticonvulsant medications and bone mineral density. *Endocr Pract*. 2012:1-22.

37. Arora E, Singh H, Gupta YK. Impact of antiepileptic drugs on bone health: Need for monitoring, treatment, and prevention strategies. *J Family Med Prim Care*. 2016;5:248-253.

38. Miziak B, Blaszczyk B, Chroscinska-Krawczyk M, et al. The problem of osteoporosis in epileptic patients taking antiepilep-tic drugs. *Expert Opin Drug Saf*. 2014;13:935-946.

39. Shen C, Chen F, Zhang Y, Guo Y, Ding M. Association between use of antiepileptic drugs and fracture risk: a systematic review and meta-analysis. *Bone*. 2014;64:246-253.

40. Fan HC, Lee HS, Chang KP. The impact of anti-epileptic drugs on growth and bone metabolism. *Int J Mol Sci*. 2016;17(8). doi: 10.3390/ijms17081242.

41. Court-Brown, CM, Clement ND, Duckworth AD, Biant LC, McQueen MM. The changing epidemiology of fall-related fractures in adults. *Injury*. 2017;48(4):819-824.

42. Kanis JA, Burlet N, Cooper C, et al. European guidance for the diagnosis and management of osteoporosis in postmenopausal women. *Osteoporos Int*. 2008;19(4):399-428.

43. Kanis JA, Oden A, Johnell O, et al. The use of clinical risk factors enhances the performance of BMD in the prediction of hip and osteoporotic fractures in men and women. *Osteoporos Int*. 2007;18(8):1033-1046.

44. Lewiecki EM, Compston JE, Miller PD, et al. Official Positions for FRAX® Bone Mineral Density and FRAX® simplification from Joint Official Positions Development Conference of the International Society for Clinical Densitometry and International Osteoporosis Foundation on FRAX®. *J Clin Densitom*. 2011;14(3):226-236.

45. FRAX®: Fracture Risk Assessment Tool Web site. http://www.sheffield.ac.uk/FRAX/. Accessed May 30, 2017.

46. Siris ES, Baim S, Nattiv A. Primary care use of FRAX: absolute fracture risk assessment in postmenopausal women and older men. *Postgrad Med*. 2010;122(1):82-90.

47. Leslie WD, Lix LM, Johansson H, et al. Spine-hip discordance and fracture risk assessment: a physician-friendly FRAX enhancement. *Osteoporos Int*. 2011;22(3):839-847.

48. Johansson H, Kanis JA, Oden A, et al. Impact of femoral neck and lumbar spine BMD discordance on FRAX probabilities in women: a meta-analysis of international cohorts. *Calcif Tissue Int*. 2014;95:428-435.

49. Leslie WD, Lix LM, Johansson H, Oden A, McCloskey E, Kanis JA, Manitoba Bone Density Program. Does osteoporosis therapy invalidate FRAX for fracture prediction? *J Bone Miner Res*. 2012;27(6):1243-1251.

50. He H, Liu Y, Tian Q, et al. Relationship of sarcopenia and body composition with osteoporosis. *Osteoporos Int*. 2016;27:473-482.

51. Shapses SA, Pop LC, Wang Y. Obesity is a concern for bone health with aging. *Nutrition Research*. 2017;39:1-13.

52. Papaioannou A, Morin S, Cheung AM, et al. 2010 clinical practice guidelines for the diagnosis and management of osteoporosis in Canada: summary. *CMAJ*. 2010;182(17):1864-1873.

53. Khamis S, Carmeli E. A new concept for measuring leg length discrepancy. *J Orthop*. 2017;14:276-280.

5

Diagnosis: Fracture Types, Measuring Bone Mass, Tests for Secondary Causes, and Other Methods of Skeletal Assessment

Definition of Osteoporosis

The definition from the NIH Consensus Development Panel is that osteoporosis is a skeletal disorder characterized by compromised bone strength predisposing a person to an increased risk of fracture. Bone strength primarily reflects the integration of bone density and bone quality. Bone density is expressed as grams of mineral per area (dual-energy x-ray absorptiometry) or volume and is determined by peak bone mass and the amount of bone loss. Bone quality refers to architecture, turnover, damage accumulation (eg, microfractures) and mineralization. A fracture occurs when a failure-inducing force is applied to an osteoporotic bone. Osteoporosis is a significant risk factor for fracture.[1]

Making the Diagnosis of Osteoporosis

Table 5.1 shows the World Health Organization (WHO) definitions of low bone mass and osteoporosis using bone mineral density (BMD) T-score criteria.[2,3]

The cutoff of -2.5 was selected to make the prevalence of osteoporosis at the hip, spine, or forearm in postmenopausal women approximately equal to the lifetime risk of fracture at the hip, spine, or forearm.

The original WHO classification applied to Caucasian postmenopausal women and therefore, may not apply as well to other ethnic groups. In addition, the WHO definition does not distinguish between

TABLE 5.1 — WHO Definitions of Osteoporosis

Status	SD of Patient BMD From That of Young Normal Adult (T-score)
Normal	T-score $\geq$-1.0 SD
Low bone mass	-2.5 SD < T-score <-1.0 SD
Osteoporosis	T-score $\leq$-2.5 SD
Severe osteoporosis	T-score $\leq$-2.5 plus one or more fragility fractures

Report of a WHO Study Group. *World Health Organ Tech Rep Ser.* 1994;843:1-129 and Kanis JA, et al. *J Bone Miner Res.* 1994;9(8):1137-1141.

postmenopausal osteoporosis and other causes of osteoporosis. The consensus guidelines below from the International Society of Clinical Densitometry (ISCD) discuss sites for diagnosis, databases, and the use of T-scores and Z-scores:

- In postmenopausal women and men >50 years of age, the diagnostic T-score definitions are applied to measurements taken by central DXA of the lumbar spine, total hip, femoral neck, and 1/3 radius.[4,5]
- The lowest T-score of the lumbar spine, hip (total hip and femoral neck), and 1/3 radius gives the diagnostic classification.[4,5]
- A Caucasian (non–race-adjusted) database is used in the calculation of T-scores for women in all ethnic groups and Z-scores are calculated based on a self-reported ethnicity database, if available.[4,5]
- Use a uniform (non-raced adjusted) female reference for men of all ethnic groups for a T-score.[5]
- Manufacturers should continue to use NHANES III data as the reference stand for femoral neck and total hip T-scores.[4,5]
- Manufacturers should continue to use their own databases for the lumbar spine as the reference standard for T-scores.[4,5]
- T-scores should not be applied to premenopausal women, men <50 years of age, or children. In this group, Z-scores are preferred.[4]
  – A Z-score ≤-2.0 is considered below the expected range for age.
  – A Z-score >-2.0 is considered to be within the expected range for age.
- Z-scores should be population specific where adequate reference data exist. For the purpose of Z-score calculation, the patient's self-reported ethnicity should be used.[4]

Fragility Fractures

The diagnosis of osteoporosis can also be made on the presence of a low-trauma (fragility or insufficiency) fracture alone.[6] A fragility fracture is usually defined as a fracture occurring after a fall from a standing height or less. Fractures of the hands, feet, nose, and skull are usually not considered to be fragility fractures. The presence of one fragility fracture is strongly predictive of future fragility fractures (**Figure 5.1**).[7-9] However, in older adults, high-trauma nonspinal fractures are also associated with low BMD.[10]

■ Spine Fractures

Spinal compression fractures are the most common type of fragility fracture and begin to increase in women at the time of menopause with the loss of trabecular bone. The long-term sequelae of compression fractures are height loss, diminished quality of life, restrictive pulmonary disease, increased risk of future fractures, and increased mortality.[11] Morphometric vertebral fracture prevalence is highest in Scandinavia (26%) and is lowest in Eastern Europe (18%). The prevalence in North American Caucasian women is 20% to 24% for ages ≥50. Vertebral fractures are approximately four times higher in white men and women than in Blacks.[12]

■ Hip Fractures

Hip fractures are the second most common fragility fracture. Most hip fractures occur from a standing height, are symptomatic, and are diagnosed radiologically. Approximately one half of individuals are permanently incapacitated after a hip fracture and approximately 20% require long-term nursing home care. There is up to 30% increased mortality within the first year after a hip fracture.[13,14] The presence of a hip fracture confers a 2.3-fold increased relative risk of a future hip fracture and 2.5-fold increased relative risk of a vertebral compression fracture.[7,9]

FIGURE 5.1 — Prevalent Vertebral Fractures Increases Future Fracture Risk

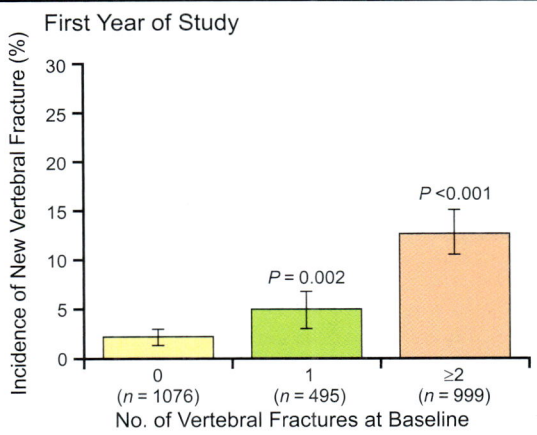

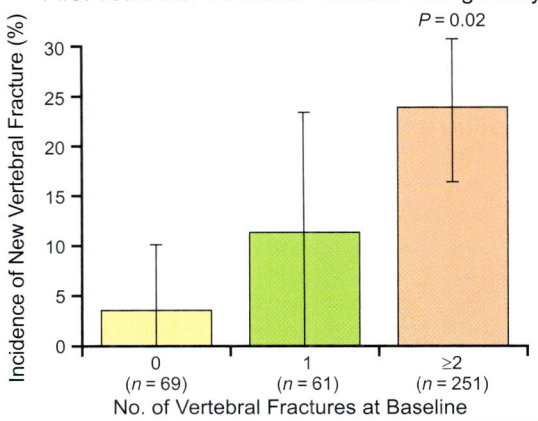

Incidence is based on Kaplan-Meier estimates of the survival function. Error bars indicate 95% CI.

Lindsay R, et al. *JAMA*. 2001;285(3):320-323.

■ Wrist Fractures

Wrist fractures are the third most common type of fragility fracture. Most wrist fractures occur with a fall from a standing height and landing on an outstretched hand. Wrist fractures are complicated by temporary pain and disability but may be complicated by long-term problems such as reflex sympathetic dystrophy.[15]

Evaluating Secondary Causes of Osteoporosis

The BMD diagnosis of low bone mass or osteoporosis does not give specific information about the timing of bone loss or the cause of bone loss. An individual with low BMD may have never achieved a high bone mass (ie, low peak bone mass) or may have had a reason to lose BMD other than osteoporosis. Most young adults with low bone mass do not have osteoporosis, given an absence of ongoing microarchitectural deterioration.

Secondary causes of osteoporosis are believed to be present in approximately 30% of cases in postmenopausal women. These may often be identified by a careful history and physical examination, but additional testing should be considered in all subjects. In men, common causes of low BMD are hypogonadism, alcoholism, and use of glucocorticoids (**Table 4.1**). **Table 5.2** lists laboratory tests that may be checked for the evaluation of secondary causes.[16]

A strategy of measuring serum calcium, a serum thyroid-stimulating hormone (TSH), serum intact parathyroid hormone level (iPTH), a 24-hour urine calcium, and a 25-OH vitamin D level is relatively cost-effective way to rule out secondary causes.[17] When prompted by other clinical or laboratory clues, other testing may include measurement of IgA anti-tissue transglutaminase antibodies and IgA endomysial antibody to rule out celiac sprue, an immunofixation electrophoresis, and free light chains to rule out a myeloma or monoclonal

TABLE 5.2 — Laboratory Evaluation of Secondary Causes of Decreased Bone Mass

Test	Diagnosis Ruled In or Ruled Out
Serum protein electrophoresis/complete blood count	Multiple myeloma
Serum calcium and phosphorus	Hyperparathyroidism
Serum intact parathyroid hormone	Hyperparathyroidism
Serum creatinine	Renal failure
Liver enzymes	Liver failure
24-Hour urine-free cortisol or dexamethasone suppression test	Cushing's syndrome
Thyroid-stimulating hormone	Hyperthyroidism
Follicle-stimulating hormone	Menopause
Free testosterone	Male hypogonadism
Urine calcium/creatinine ratio and/or 24-hour urine for calcium excretion	Hypercalciuria
25-Monohydroxy vitamin D_3 and alkaline phosphatase	Vitamin D deficiency or osteomalacia
Antitransglutaminase antibodies	Celiac sprue

Boulware DW, Heudebert GR. *Lippincott's Primary Care Rheumatology*. Philadelphia, PA: Wolters Kluwer/Lippincott Williams & Wilkins; 2011.

5

gammopathy. Tests of adrenal function should be performed if Cushing's disease is suspected and, in men, measurement of testosterone and gonadotrophins should be considered.

DXA for Measuring BMD

Bone mineral density (BMD) is one component of bone strength. Dual-energy x-ray absorptiometry (DXA) measures BMD and is used for the purpose of diagnosing osteoporosis, assessing fracture risk, and monitoring changes in BMD over time. DXA uses ionizing radiation, with photon beams of two different energy levels to measure bone mineral content in grams and bone area in square centimeters. Therefore, DXA measures BMD as an areal density (grams per square centimeter). This technology quantitates BMD by separating bone mineral from soft tissue.

Advantages of DXA include:
- Good accuracy and precision
- Low radiation dose
- DXA values form the basis for the diagnostic classification of osteoporosis
- Patients shown to benefit from pharmacologic intervention in most clinical trials were selected by DXA-measured BMD.

Reporting Bone Mass and Definition of Osteoporosis

Two ways of evaluating/reporting bone density based on BMD measurements are available. The T-score is the number of standard deviations (SDs) from the normal young adult mean value; the Z-score is the number of SDs from the normal mean value for age-, race-, and sex-matched control subjects. T-scores are used for diagnosis of osteoporosis in postmenopausal women and men ≥ age 50, but should not be used for this purpose in younger individuals.[4]

■ **Reference Values**

The reference populations for DXA scanning are based on studies of healthy subjects without known metabolic bone disease or fractures who are not taking medications known to impact on bone physiology. T-scores at the spine are calculated from the manufacturers' healthy young adult reference databases and may vary according to the instrument used. T-scores in the hip are based on the National Health and Nutrition Examination Survey (NHANES) III white database for individuals aged 20 to 29. In the United States, the T-score is based on a white data base (non-race adjusted), while Z-scores are calculated based on a self-reported ethnicity database. For T-scores, both males and females are compared to a uniform non-race adjusted female reference database.[4] See the section above (*Making the Diagnosis of Osteoporosis*) for a discussion related to the use of Z-scores in premenopausal women and men under the age of 50. Recommendations exist related to densitometry in pediatrics.[5]

Bone Mass and Fracture Risk

Currently, DXA is the gold standard technology for assessing fracture risk because BMD and bone strength are strongly correlated. Bone mass is said to account for approximately 60% to 80% of the variation in the ultimate strength of bone tissue. Studies confirm that reduced bone mass, irrespective of the site of measurement, is correlated with an increased risk for future fracture. The relative risk of fracture increases approximately by 2-fold for each one standard deviation decrease in bone mineral density below the age-adjusted mean BMD. Although peripheral densitometry is predictive of hip and spine fractures and may be suitable for screening, hip and vertebral fractures are more strongly associated with bone density of the directly measured proximal femur and vertebrae, respectively. Compared with serum cholesterol measurements, bone density is a better predictor for osteoporosis than hypercholesterolemia is for cardiovascular disease.

Recommended Sites for DXA Diagnosis

The ISCD recommends that DXA measurements for diagnosis be done at several sites: the PA spine and proximal femur (total hip and femoral neck) in all patients, and the forearm in patients for whom hip and/or spine BMD cannot be measured, or where there is hyperparathyroidism or patients who are above the weight limit of the scanning table.[4]

■ **Spine Sites**

For spine BMD measurement, use all evaluable vertebrae, L1-L4, from posteroanterior view (**Figure 5.2**). Vertebral bodies that are structurally changed by fracture, osteophytes, or scoliosis or overlying artifacts should be excluded. The reported spine BMD value should be obtained from more than one vertebra. If that is not possible, BMD diagnosis should be based on a different skeletal site. The lateral spine should not be used for diagnosis of osteoporosis.

■ **Hip Sites**

Using either hip, DXA BMD measurements are obtained at the femoral neck and total hip (**Figure 5.3**). Some DXA machines have the capability of performing dual hip scans.

■ **Forearm Sites**

For forearm BMD measurements, use the one-third (33%) radius of the nondominant arm. Other forearm sites are not recommended for diagnosis or follow-up (**Figure 5.4**).

How to Interpret a DXA Scan

The interpretation of the data is similar regardless of the manufacturer of the DXA equipment. To improve accuracy and precision, the same machine should be used for repeat testing. Certification for reading and interpretation of DXA scans is available from the ISCD for both clinicians/researchers (Certified Clinical Densitometrist™®) and technologists (Certified Bone Densitometry Technologist™®). In addition, accreditation of DXA facilities is also available from the ISCD (www.iscd.org).

▣ General Analysis

Are the patient's demographics correct? This is essential for age-matched comparisons and to assure the use of the correct Z-score database. It is helpful to have a patient information sheet that a patient fills out that documents pertinent demographics and clinical history (**Figure 5.5**).

■ Lumbar Spine Analysis

In assessing the lumbar spine scan, the following should be considered (**Figure 5.2**):

- Are any artifacts present on the scan within the field of interest?
- Is the patient straight on the table with an approximately equal amount of soft tissue on either side of the spine? Spine scans are usually completed with the patient's legs up on a block. The spine should not be rotated.
- Are the vertebrae, T12-L5, and the iliac crests clearly visible to assist with the identification of spinal levels? The top of the iliac crest usually defines the L4-L5 interspace.
- Approximately 17% of individuals will not have 5 lumbar vertebral bodies or the ribs on T12, therefore, the possibility of segmentation variations should be considered.[18]
- It is recommended that vertebral levels are numbered from the bottom up from what is designated the L4-L5 interspace. It is especially important to make sure that the same vertebral levels are being scanned in follow-up exams.
- Are the intervertebral spaces correctly marked?

FIGURE 5.2 — Lumbar Spine DXA Scan

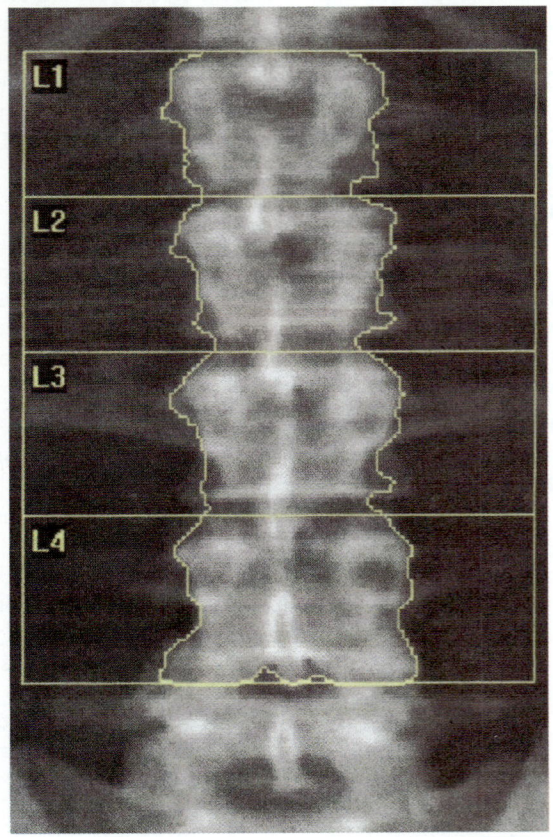

DXA scan of L1-L4 in the lumbar spine of a 52-year-old, 70-inch tall, 160-pound Caucasian man. The iliac crest is visible and the lowest ribs are present at T12. The edge detection and the intervertebral spaces are correctly marked. There are no artifacts within the region of interest scanned. In a 52-year-old man, it is correct to report a T-score, and a male database is used in the calculation of the T-score and the Z-score.

Continued

FIGURE 5.2 — *Continued*

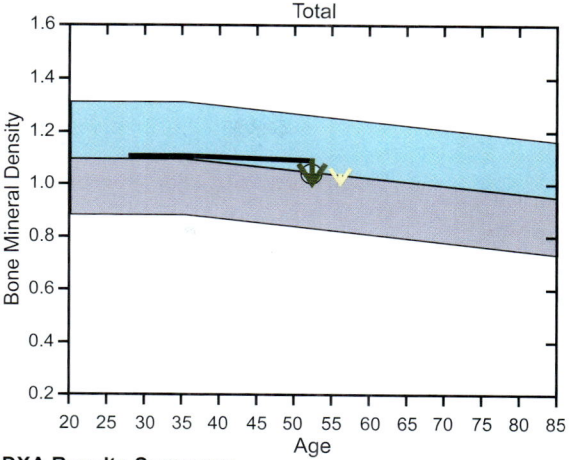

DXA Results Summary:

Region	Area (cm²)	BMC (g)	BMD (g/cm²)	T-score	PR (%)	Z-score	AM (%)
L1	14.83	13.73	0.926	-1.3	86	-1.0	90
L2	15.81	16.47	1.042	-0.5	95	-0.1	99
L3	17.05	18.20	1.067	-0.3	97	0.1	101
L4	19.82	21.58	1.089	0.0	100	0.4	104
Total	**67.51**	**69.99**	**1.037**	**-0.5**	**95**	**-0.1**	**99**

Total BMD CV 1.0%, ACF = 1.012, BCF = 0.987, TH = 7.025
WHO classification: Normal
Fracture risk: Not increased

The reference graph shows the BMD of a man, age 52, that is 0.5 standard deviations below the young mean adult value (T-score) *(large green arrow)* and 0.1 standard deviation below the age-matched control (Z-score) *(small yellow arrow)*. The bars on the graph are ± 2 standard deviations. The middle line between the bars in the graph is the average BMD for age. Based on this site alone, the diagnosis would be normal BMD.

FIGURE 5.3 — DXA Scan of the Hip

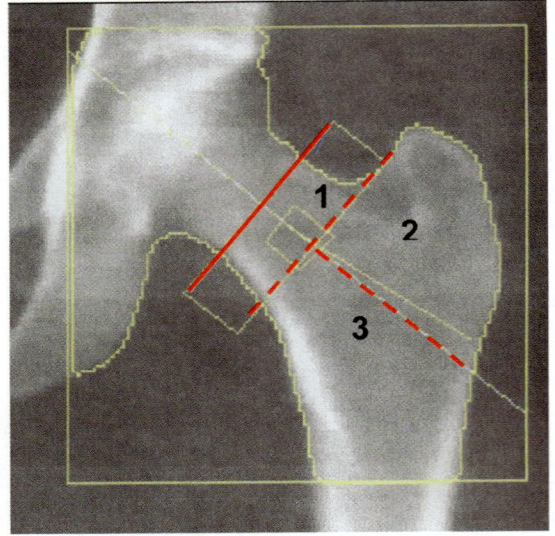

DXA scan of the hip in a 49-year-old, 60-inch tall, 135-pound postmenopausal Caucasian woman. The femoral neck region of interest is area 1. The total hip region of interest represents the sum of area 1 (femoral neck) + 2 (trochanter) + 3 (intertrochanteric/shaft) regions of interest. The shaft of the femur is straight and the hip is internally rotated. There are no artifacts within the region of interest scanned. In scanning a female, a female reference database is used. Because the patient is postmenopausal, it is correct to use a T-score in reporting the BMD.

Continued

- Is the edge detection correct (ie, the outlined boundaries between bone and soft tissue)?
- Is there scoliosis? If so, has this been considered in the analysis?
- Vertebral density and area generally increases going from L1 to L4 and contiguous vertebral bodies are within one standard deviation of each other. If there a marked difference in the bone density and/or area of different vertebrae, this

FIGURE 5.3 — *Continued*

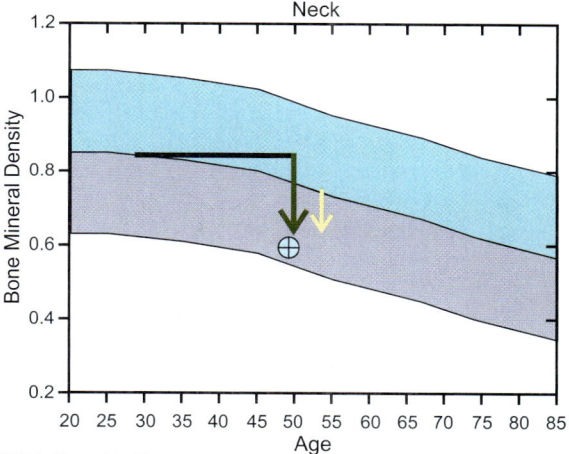

DXA Results Summary:

Region	Area (cm²)	BMC (g)	BMD (g/cm²)	T-score	PR (%)	Z-score	AM (%)
Neck	4.40	2.61	0.594	-2.3	70	-1.6	77
Total	30.52	22.42	0.735	-1.7	78	-1.3	83

Total BMD CV 1.0%, ACF = 1.009, BCF = 0.99, TH = 6.423
WHO classification: Osteopenia

The reference graph shows the femoral neck BMD of a woman, age 49, that is 2.3 standard deviations below the young mean adult value (T-score) *(large green arrow)* and 1.6 standard deviation below the age-matched control (Z-score) *(small yellow arrow)*. The bars on the graph are ±2 standard deviations. The middle line between the bars in the graph is the average BMD for age. Based on this site alone, the diagnosis would be low bone mass (osteopenia).

may indicate vertebral fractures and/or ectopic calcification secondary to disk degeneration, the presence of osteophytes, or calcified vessels or aorta. Check with anteroposterior and lateral radiographs of the lumbar and thoracic spine or consider ordering a vertebral fracture assessment (VFA).

FIGURE 5.4 — DXA Scan of the Wrist

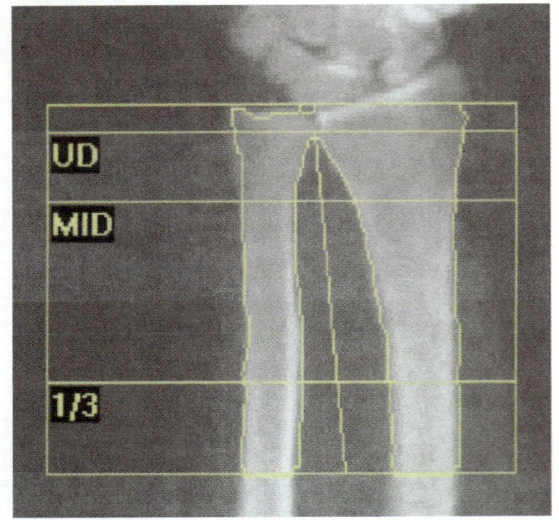

DXA scan of the forearm in a 71-year-old, 59-inch tall, 143-pound Caucasian woman. The 1/3 radius (33% radius) site is reported. There are no artifacts within the region of interest scanned. In scanning a female, a female reference database is used.

Continued

Interpreting the Data

Compare the BMD of L1 through L4 with the young adult score (T-score) or the value for age-matched subjects (Z-score), depending on age to make a diagnosis. (**Figure 5.2**). The data are also used to decide on appropriate therapy, often using absolute fracture risk algorithms such as FRAX®,[19] monitor response to treatment, and determine the frequency of repeat testing.

■ **Hip Analysis**

The two areas of interest recommended for reporting by the ISCD are shown in **Figure 5.3** and are the femoral neck and total hip (the total hip is the sum of

FIGURE 5.4 — *Continued*

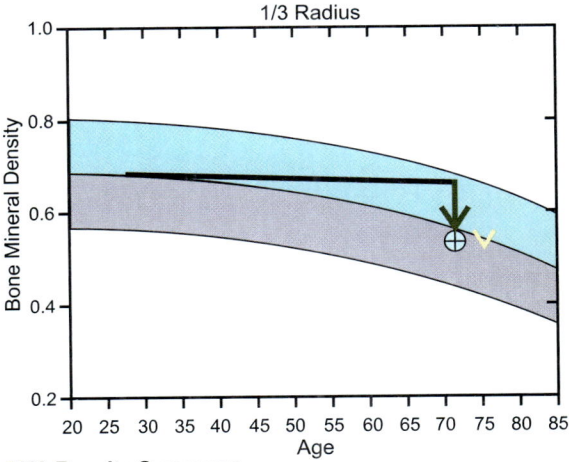

DXA Results Summary:

Region	Area (cm²)	BMC (g)	BMD (g/cm²)	T-score	PR (%)	Z-score	AM (%)
UD	3.45	1.14	0.329	-2.0	74	-0.4	93
MID	5.51	2.54	0.461	-2.7	76	-0.5	94
1/3	2.55	1.38	0.543	-2.5	78	-0.4	96
Total	11.51	5.06	0.439	-2.6	76	-0.5	94

Total BMD CV 1.0%, ACF = 1.009, BCF = 0.99
WHO classification: Osteoporosis
Fracture risk: High

The reference graph shows the BMD of the 1/3 radius of a woman, age 71, that is 2.5 standard deviations below the young mean adult value (T-score) *(large green arrow)* and 0.4 standard deviation below the age-matched control (Z-score) *(small yellow arrow)*. The bars on the graph are ± 2 standard deviations. The middle line between the bars in the graph is the average BMD for age. Based on this site alone, the diagnosis would be osteoporosis.

FIGURE 5.5 — Example of a DXA Facility Patient Questionnaire

⌊∃ Osteoporosis Prevention and Treatment Clinic

Office use only
Place sticker here

Name _____
M.R. # _____

IS THERE ANY CHANCE THAT YOU ARE PREGNANT?   □ No □ Yes

1. Have you had an x-ray with barium, contrast, or a nuclear medicine test within the last 72 hours? □ No □ Yes

2. What is your current age? _____

3. How much height have you lost since age 25? _____ (inches) Weight _____ (pounds)
   _____ (inches) □ None □ Don't know

4. What is your ethnicity/race? (Please select one)
   □ Caucasian/White   □ Native American Indian   □ Asian
   □ African-American/Black   □ Hispanic   □ Pacific Islander   □ Multiracial

5. What is your sex?   □ Male   □ Female

6. If you are a **FEMALE**,....
   □ No □ Yes   Are you postmenopausal and/or stopped having menstrual periods?
   □ No □ Yes   Have you had your uterus removed?
   □ No □ Yes   Have you had **both** ovaries removed?

7. Do you **CURRENTLY** take steroids (Prednisone, Cortisol, Deltasone, or Medrol) by **mouth**?   □ No □ Yes
   (Do **not** answer "yes" for inhaled or poorly absorbed steroids used for GI purposes)

8. Have you broken (fractured) any bones after the age of 50?   □ No □ Yes

9. If **YES**, check the type of fracture that you have had after the age of 50 (Please check all that apply):

□ Spine/back   □ Rib   □ Shoulder   □ Foot

□ Wrist/forearm   □ Hip   □ Ankle   □ Other _____

10. Has your mother or father had a hip fracture after the age of 50?   □ No   □ Yes   □ Don't know

(Do not answer if you are adopted. Do not answer "yes" for hip replacements for non-fracture reasons like arthritis)

11. Are you currently a cigarette smoker?   □ No   □ Yes

12. **Do you drink alcohol every day?**   □ No   □ Yes

If yes, do you drink ≥3 cans of beer and/or ≥3 glasses of wine (1 glass = ½ cup) and/or   □ No   □ Yes

≥3 shots of hard liquor per day?

13. Do you **USUALLY** need to use your arms to assist yourself in standing up from a chair?   □ No   □ Yes

14. Have you had surgery on your lower back and/or a vertebroplasty or a kyphoplasty?   □ No   □ Yes

(injection of cement in your spine after a compression fracture)

Continued

FIGURE 5.5 — *Continued*

15. Have you taken in the **PAST** OR are you **NOW** taking any of the following bone medications?

	NEVER Taken	Taken in the **PAST**	**NOW** Taking	If taken in the **PAST** OR **NOW** taking, for how long?
Actonel (risedronate)	☐	☐	☐	_____ years
Boniva (ibandronate)	☐	☐	☐	_____ years
Miacalcin (calcitonin spray)	☐	☐	☐	_____ years
Estrogen (hormone therapy)	☐	☐	☐	_____ years
Evista (raloxifene)	☐	☐	☐	_____ years
Forteo (PTH)	☐	☐	☐	_____ years
Fosamax (alendronate)	☐	☐	☐	_____ years
Reclast (zoledronic acid)	☐	☐	☐	_____ years
Prolia (denosumab)	☐	☐	☐	_____ years

16. Do you have hyperparathyroidism? (4 overactive small glands near your thyroid)
(**NOT THYROID PROBLEMS**)   ☐ No ☐ Yes

17. Do you have any of these other medical problems?–If so, check the box:

- ☐ No ☐ Yes Lupus
- ☐ No ☐ Yes Rheumatoid arthritis (only if a doctor has diagnosed, don't answer "yes" for osteoarthritis, gout, or pain syndromes like fibromyalgia)
- ☐ No ☐ Yes Transplant If **YES**, type _____
- ☐ No ☐ Yes Asthma
- ☐ No ☐ Yes COPD (emphysema)
- ☐ No ☐ Yes Anorexia nervosa or bulimia nervosa
- ☐ No ☐ Yes Prostate cancer
- ☐ No ☐ Yes Breast cancer
- ☐ No ☐ Yes Kidney failure
- ☐ No ☐ Yes Crohn's disease or ulcerative colitis

18. *Are you interested in being contacted about Osteoporosis Research at UAB?* ☐ No ☐ Yes

5

the femoral neck, the trochanter, and the intertrochanteric regions of interest). Additional considerations include:

- Are any artifacts present within the region of interest?
- The shaft of the femur should be straight the hip should be internally rotated so a minimal amount of lesser trochanter is visible. Variations in rotation of the hip can particularly affect the BMD of the femoral neck.[20]
- The placement of the region of interest box/triangle for the total proximal femur will vary with the manufacturer.
- The placement of the femoral neck box also varies by manufacturer. In a Hologic scan, the femoral neck box is anchored to the greater trochanter. On a GE Lunar scan, the femoral neck box is at the narrowest area of the femoral neck. Check with the manufacturer's instruction manual related to the correct positioning of analysis lines and the region of interest boxes/triangles.
- It is important to make sure that nothing else, such as the ischium or trochanter, is in the femoral neck box. There are ways to manually omit other bone that is within the femoral neck box.

Interpreting the Data

- The bone in the femoral neck is composed of relatively more cortical bone than in the total hip region of interest. (**Figure 5.3**).
- Comparisons of BMD in the above regions are made with the young adult score (T-score) and that of an age-matched subject (Z-score) to make a diagnosis. The data are also used to decide on appropriate therapy, often using absolute fracture risk algorithms such as FRAX®[19] (the femoral neck BMD is used in the FRAX® calculation), monitor response to treatment, and determine the frequency of repeat testing.

■ **Forearm Analysis**

The area of interest is shown in **Figure 5.4**:

- The nondominant arm is scanned unless there is arthritis or a fracture.
- A positioning device is used.
- Are any artifacts present within the region of interest scanned?
- Check with the manufacturer instructions related to the correct positioning of the region of interest boxes and whether a wrist positioner should be used.

Interpreting the Data

Comparison of BMD in the 1/3 region is made with the young adult score (T-score) and that of an age-matched subject (Z-score) to make a diagnosis (**Figure 5.4**). The data are also used to decide on appropriate therapy, often using absolute fracture risk algorithms, such as FRAX®,[19] monitor response to treatment, and determine the frequency of repeat testing.

■ **Assessment of Change**

It is important to make sure that follow-up scans are completed on the same DXA scanner or a cross-calibrated scanner. For many reasons, it is not possible to make comparisons of scans made on DXA scanners from different manufacturers or on scanners that have not been cross calibrated. The ISCD recommends using the lumbar spine and total hip as the sites to gauge change in BMD. It is recommended that each DXA facility determine their short-term precision for each anatomical site by completing a short-term precision study[4]:

- Comparisons between interval scans are best made by determining the change in g/sq cm and comparing to the least significant change at the specific site (using the precision error and the desired confidence interval).
- A change in BMD is significant if the change is equal to or greater than the least significant change (either positive or negative).

- The compare feature should be used in evaluating follow-up scans to assure that positioning and analogous regions of interest are compared.

■ DXA Quality and Quality Assurance

It has increasingly been documented that there are problems with DXA scan acquisition, analysis, interpretation, and reporting.[21] A review of DXA images at an Italian university found that 90% of exams and reports had one or more errors.[22] Approximately 79% of the errors were related to data analysis, 12% were related to patient positioning, 7% were to related to the presence of artifacts, and 2% were related to incorrect demographics.[22]

To assure DXA quality, each DXA center should have a quality control program[4]:

- Each facility should comply with local, state, and national radiation safety regulations.
- Internal or external calibration assures that the machine is functioning correctly.
- Scanning a spine phantom assures that the results are stable over time.
- The ISCD recommends at least once a week phantom scans.
- The calibration and phantom scans should be plotted and reviewed regularly to assure that the machine is operating correctly.

Each facility should have standard operating procedures written.

Best practices have been published which list minimal quality standards for scan acquisition, analysis, interpretation, and reporting.[23] **Table 5.3** shows these performance measures. It is recommended that DXA pay for performance measures be developed which would recognize fulfillment of quality measures, certification of technologists and clinicians, and accreditation of DXA facilities.

TABLE 5.3 — DXA Best Practices

Scan Acquisition and Analysis

1.1. At least one practicing DXA technologist, and preferably all, has a valid certification in bone densitometry.

1.2. Each DXA technologist has access to the manufacturer's manual of technical standards and applies these standards for BMD measurement.

1.3. Each DXA facility has detailed standard operating procedures for DXA performance that are updated when appropriate and available for review by all key personnel.

1.4. The DXA facility must comply with all applicable radiation safety requirements.

1.5. Spine phantom BMD measurement is performed at least once weekly to document stability operating of DXA performance over time. BMD values must be maintained within a tolerance of $\pm$ 1.5%, with a defined ongoing monitoring plan that defines a correction approach when the tolerance has been exceeded.

1.6. Each DXA technologist has performed in vivo precision assessment according to standard methods and the facility LSC has been calculated.

1.7. The LSC for each DXA technologist should not exceed 5.3% for the lumbar spine, 5.0% for the total proximal femur, and 6.9% for the femoral neck.

Interpretation and Reporting

2.1. At least one practicing DXA interpreter, and preferably all, has a valid certification in bone densitometry.

2.2. The DXA manufacturer and model are noted on the report.

2.3. The DXA report includes a statement regarding scan factors that may adversely affect acquisition/analysis quality and artifacts/confounders, if present.

2.4. The DXA report identifies the skeletal site, region of interest, and body side for each technically valid BMD measurement.

2.5. There is a single diagnosis reported for each patient, not a different diagnosis for each skeletal site measured.

2.6. A fracture risk assessment tool is used appropriately.

2.7. When reporting differences in BMD with serial measurements, only those changes that meet or exceed the LSC are reported as a change.

Lewiecki EM, et al. *J Clin Densitom*. 2016;19(2):127-140.

- **Reporting DXA Scans**

    The ISCD has established minimum requirements for DXA reports[4]:

    - Demographics
    - Fracture risk factors including information about previous fragility fractures
    - The requesting provider
    - Indication for ordering the test
    - The name of the manufacturer and model of the instrument
    - A statement about the technical quality of the scan. If a region of interest is not valid or is excluded a statement should explain the limitation
    - BMD in g/sq cm for each site
    - The T-score and/or Z-score
    - WHO criteria for diagnosis in postmenopausal females and males > age 50
    - A statement about fracture risk, where appropriate
    - A general statement about evaluation for secondary causes may be appropriate
    - A recommendation for the necessity and timing of the next DXA exam.
    - A suggested template for DXA reporting is available at https://iscd.app.b.x.com/v/us-adult-dxa-sample-report.

Screening and Retesting for Osteoporosis

- **Screening Tests**

    Among bone measurement tests used to screen for osteoporosis central DXA of the hip and lumbar spine is the most widely used. Peripheral DXA (pDXA) of the heel or forearm may also be used. Quantitative ultrasound (QUS) of the calcaneus predicts fractures of the femoral neck, hip, and spine as effectively as DXA, but accepted diagnostic and treatment criteria for osteoporosis use DXA measurements because evaluation criteria based on QUS do not exist.

■ **At What Age Should Individuals Be Screened for Osteoporosis?**

In 2007, the ISCD proposed criteria for BMD testing (**Table 5.4**).[4] The National Osteoporosis Foundation has also written guidelines for BMD testing (**Table 4.2**).[16] The US Preventive Services Task Force (USPSTF), the National Osteoporosis Foundation (NOF), American Association of Clinical Endocrinologists (AACE),[24] and the ISCD have recommended that all women should have a measurement of BMD at the age of 65 years.[4,16,25,26] This recommendation is based on the increase in the incidence of fracture

TABLE 5.4 — Indications for Bone Mass Measurement From the International Society for Clinical Densitometry

- Women aged 65 years and older
- Postmenopausal women younger than 65 years with risk factors for osteoporosis
- Women during the menopause transition with clinical risk factors for fracture, such as:
  – Low body weight
  – Prior fracture
  – High-risk medication use
- Men aged 70 years and older
- Men younger than 70 years with clinical risk factors for fracture
- Adults who have fragility fracture
- Adults who have a disease or condition associated with low bone mass or bone loss
- Anyone being considered for pharmacologic osteoporosis therapy
- Anyone being treated for low bone mass to monitor treatment effect
- Anyone not undergoing therapy in whom evidence of bone loss would lead to treatment

Baim S, et al. *J Clin Densitom.* 2008;11(1):75-91; Cosman F, et al. *Osteoporos Int.* 2014;25:2359-2381.

that occurs after the age of 65 years. The USPSTF recommends that women <65 years of age who have a 10-year fracture risk greater than or equal to that of a 65-year old white woman should have BMD testing.[25] In contrast, the NOF, AACE, and ISCD suggest that any postmenopausal woman with multiple risk factors should be tested. The ISCD and AACE have provided additional guidelines for testing in men, premenopausal and perimenopausal women, and children.[4,26] These guidelines recommend BMD testing in patients who have diseases or are receiving drugs that are likely to cause secondary osteoporosis and in all patients with fragility fractures.

The United States Preventive Services Task Force has recommended DXA screening for all women ≥65 years of age without know risk factors or fractures.[27] DXA screening is recommended for women <65 years of age who have a 10-year fracture risk ≥ to the risk of a 65-year old white woman without additional risk factors (=9.3%). At the present time, there is no recommendation for DXA scanning in men without fractures or known secondary causes of osteoporosis. Guidelines from the National Osteoporosis Guideline Group in the United Kingdom provide criteria for obtaining a DXA scan based upon FRAX® fracture probabilities.[28,29]

■ Indications for DXA Testing From the Centers for Medicare & Medicaid Services and Follow-Up Testing

The indications for BMD testing from the United States Centers for Medicare and Medicaid Services (CMS) are shown in **Table 5.5**.[30] CMS will generally pay for a repeat DXA scan every 24 months. If the initial screening test did not detect osteoporosis, retesting can be done. A recent analysis from the Study of Osteoporotic fractures (SOF) has suggested a screening interval of around 17 years in postmenopausal women with normal BMD or mild low bone mass, 4.7 years in women with moderate low bone mass, and 1.1 years in women with severe low bone mass.[31] The best guidance related to DXA coverage issues is generally to

TABLE 5.5 — Indications for BMD Coverage From the US Centers for Medicare and Medicaid Services (CMS)

Medicare covers BMD testing for many individuals age 65 and older, including but not limited to:

- Estrogen-deficient women at clinical risk for osteoporosis
- Individuals with vertebral abnormalities
- Individuals receiving, or planning to receive, long-term glucocorticoid therapy in a daily dose ≥5 mg prednisone or equivalent for ≥3 months
- Individuals with primary hyperparathyroidism
- Individuals being monitored to assess the response or efficacy of an approved osteoporosis drug therapy

Cosman F, et al. *Osteoporos Int.* 2014;25:2359-2381.

check with the individual payer. A study in men > age 65 found that if the T-score was >-1.5. in the lumbar spine, total hip, and femoral neck on a first DXA scan, that those men were unlikely to develop osteoporosis. They recommended follow-up DXA scan in older men with T-scores ≤-1.5.[32]

■ Osteoporosis and Fracture Risk Assessment Tools

There are several risk-assessment tools that can evaluate future potential for fractures. Most of these can be used in conjunction with BMD testing to screen for osteoporosis; however, some may generate a fracture risk based on clinical risk factors alone. A general theme of fracture risk calculators is moving away from relative risk to absolute risk to quantitate fracture risk. The use of these fracture risk tools in treatment decisions is further discussed in *Chapter 9*.

- Fracture-risk algorithm (FRAX®) (www.sheffield.ac.uk/FRAX/) (see *Chapter 4*)
- Canadian Association of Radiologist and Osteoporosis Canada (CAROC) (www.osteoporosis.ca)
- Fracture Risk Calculator (FRC) (www.fore.org)

- Garvan fracture risk calculator (www.garvan .org.au)
- Qfracture (www.qfracture.org/).

Other Methods for Skeletal and Fracture Risk Assessment

BMD testing in peripheral skeletal sites, such as the heel, radius, and tibia can be done with quantitative ultrasound (QUS) and peripheral quantitative computed tomography (QCT).[33,34] QCT can also be used to measure volumetric bone density in the proximal femur and spine. The advantages of QUS devices are that they are small and portable, do not use ionizing radiation, and are less expensive than DXA. QCT uses more radiation and is more expensive than DXA. QUS data cannot be used for diagnostic classification according to World Health Organization (WHO) criteria; however, 2-D projections from femoral neck and total hip QCT may be used for the WHO diagnostic classification and are equivalent to DXA-T-scores.[5]

■ Quantitative Bone Ultrasound (QUS)

The Food and Drug Administration (FDA) has approved QUS (no radiation exposure) of bone as a predictive device of osteoporosis and related fractures (**Figure 5.6**).[35-39] The ISCD Consensus Guidelines state that the heel site is the only validated skeletal site for the use of QUS in osteoporosis management.[4] The calcaneus has a high percentage of trabecular bone, which rapidly turns over more rapidly than cortical bone; therefore the calcaneus site can be useful in monitoring changes in bone density. Ultrasound systems either use a water bath or gel as a coupling medium between the ultrasound and bone.

As with DXA technology, key issues in the clinical utility of ultrasound instruments are the reproducibility and precision of the measurements. The technology is based on the alteration of the shape, intensity, and speed of sound as it traverses a bony point of interest.

FIGURE 5.6 — Schematic Diagram of the Equipment Used for Ultrasonic Measurements

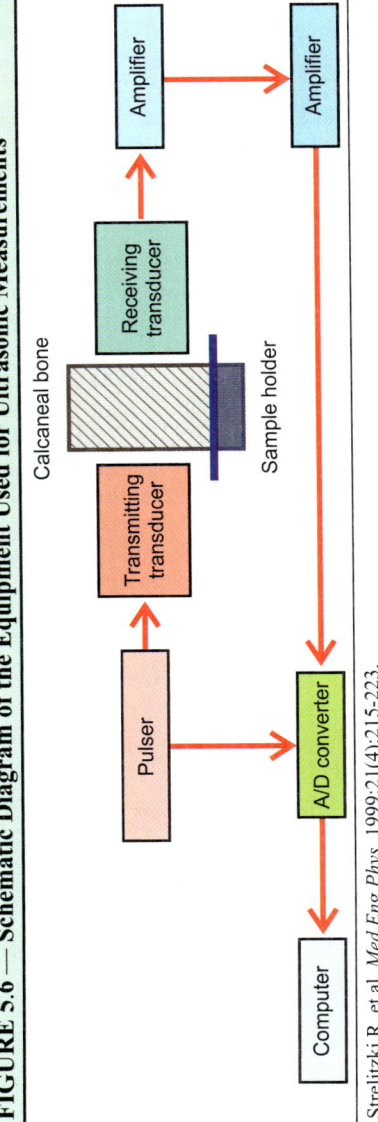

Strelitzki R, et al. *Med Eng Phys*. 1999;21(4):215-223.

5

This is quantified and serves as a qualitative measurement of the physical and mechanical property of bone, characterized by two measures:

- Speed of sound through bone (ultrasound transit velocity [SOS])
- Attenuation of sound as it passes through bone (broadband ultrasound attenuation [BUA]).

In addition, some instruments calculate measures of BUA and SOS to formulate a clinical index (quantitative ultrasound index [QUI]), usually referred to as stiffness. The site measured (calcaneus; middle third of anterior tibia) and the method of coupling (water or ultrasound gel) vary between devices.

The SOS has been shown to correlate well with BMD. BUA is influenced by structural characteristics of trabecular bone. At the heel, QUS predicts hip, spine, and global fracture risk in postmenopausal women and hip and nonvertebral fractures in men over the age of 65 years. The WHO diagnostic criteria are not applicable to QUS measurements. In a cohort of men, aged 60 to 80, for every standard deviation decrease in QUS parameters at the calcaneus, the risk of hip fracture increases 2-fold and was independent of age. QUS should not be used to monitor treatment of osteoporosis.

■ **Quantitative Computerized Tomography (QCT)**

QCT measures volumetric bone mineral density (mg/cm^3).[33,39,40] The benefits of QCT are its ability to:

- Measure volumetric BMD independent of body size
- Exclude spinal elements which contribute to BMD but do not contribute to bone strength
- Separate trabecular and cortical volumetric BMD.

A disadvantage of QCT is a significantly higher radiation dose compared with DXA. **Figure 5**.7 shows

FIGURE 5.7 — Quantitative Computerized Tomography for the Assessment of the Skeleton

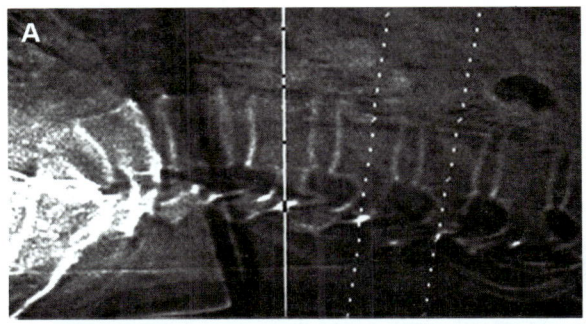

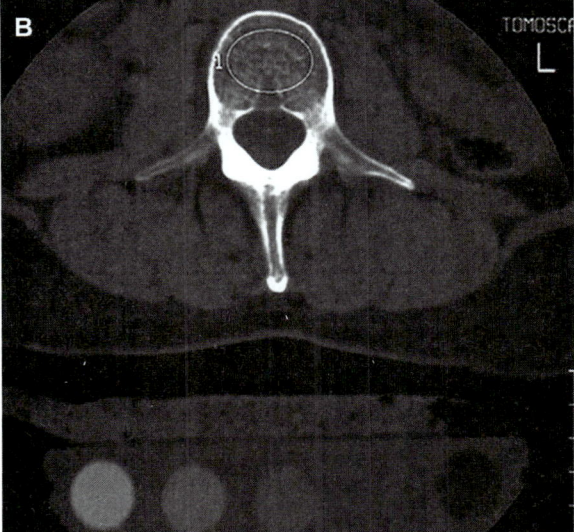

Scout image shows the location of sections obtained through the first four lumbar vertebral bodies *(A)*. Axial CT scan shows placement of an elliptic ROI to measure the volume of purely trabecular bone in a vertebral body *(B)*. The quantitative CT calibration phantom is placed under the vertebra and is used to convert Hounsfield units into milligrams per cubic centimeter of calcium hydroxyapatite.

Guglielmi G, et al. *Radiographics*. 2011;31(5):1343-1364.

the calibration phantom which is used to convert Hounsfield units to mg/cm^3 of calcium hydroxyapatite.

Spinal trabecular BMD, measured by QCT, has the same ability to predict fractures as spinal DXA in postmenopausal women. The WHO diagnostic criteria may be applied to data from 2-D projections of the femoral neck and total hip.[5] The trabecular BMD of the lumbar spine, measured by QCT can be used to monitor disease, age, and treatment-related changes.

■ Vertebral Fracture Assessment (VFA)

Vertebral fractures may be asymptomatic and it is estimated that only one in three vertebral fractures are symptomatic. Vertebral fractures can be identified using lateral x-rays of the thoracic and lumbar spine or vertebral fracture assessment (VFA) on lateral images obtained by DXA (**Figure 5.8**). Indications for vertebral imaging as outlined from the Clinician's Guide to Prevention and Treatment of Osteoporosis by the National Osteoporosis Foundation and the ISCD are shown in **Table 5.6**.[16]

The presence of vertebral fractures, a greater number of prevalent vertebral fractures, and the more severe the vertebral fractures, the greater the risk there is of a future fracture. A study has shown that the presence of one or more prevalent vertebral fractures increases the risk of further fracture 5-fold during the first year of observation compared with those subjects without prevalent vertebral fractures (relative risk [RR] 5:1).[8]

Three patterns of vertebral deformation are recognized in a VFA[41] (**Figures 5.9**):
- Wedge
- Biconcave
- Crush.

A vertebral deformation score has been proposed that can be used in longitudinal studies to quantify objectively the progress of the condition and/or response to treatment.[41] The anterior, middle, and posterior heights of the vertebrae are measured, and the fracture can be then classified as follows (**Figure 5**.9):

- *Mildly depressed (grade 1)*: 20% to 25% decrease in anterior, middle, and/or posterior height and/or reduction in 10% to 20% of the area
- *Moderately deformed (grade 2)*: 25% to 40% reduction in the height and/or a reduction in area of 20% to 40%
- *Severely deformed (grade 3)*: >40% reduction in any height and area.

It is important to note that conditions other than osteoporosis may result in vertebral deformity, including Scheuermann's disease, osteoarthritis, and some cancers. These deformities can only reliably be diagnosed on spine X-rays, so if other etiologies are suspected on DXA-based VFA, conventional X-rays should be performed to establish the cause.

■ Trabecular Bone Score

The trabecular bone score is approved as a methodology to evaluate bone microarchitecture (**Figure 5**.10).[42-44] Using DXA images, the trabecular bone score quantifies trabecular bone texture and a correlation has been shown between bone microarchitecture and fracture risk, which is independent of BMD. The TBS score can be factored into the FRAX® fracture risk assessment calculation.[45]

FIGURE 5.8 — Vertebral Fracture Assessment (VFA)

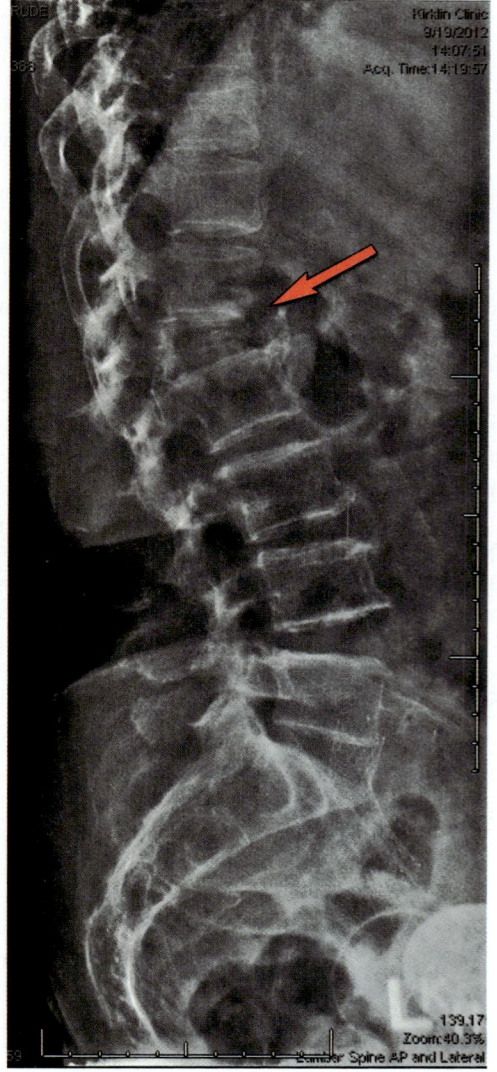

Continued

FIGURE 5.8 — *Continued*

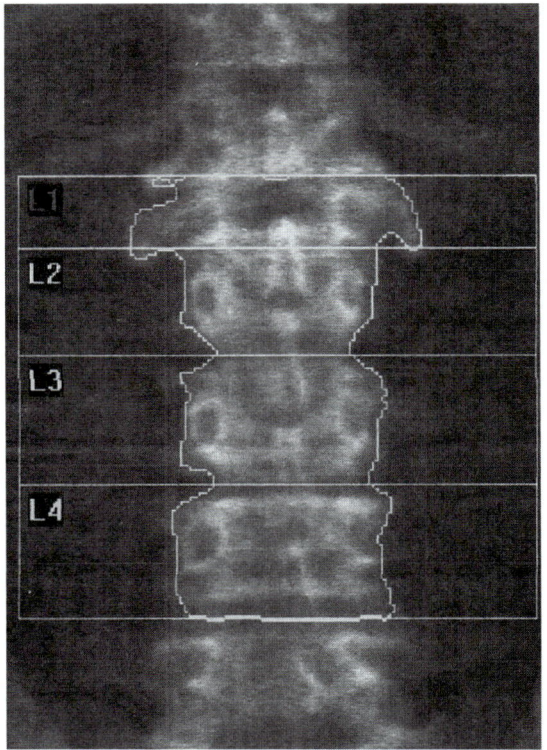

5

VFA showing an L1 fracture *(left)*. The lumbar spine radiograph *(above)* also shows the L1 fracture. According to the Genant semi-quantitative criteria, this would be classified as a grade III wedge fracture.

TABLE 5.6 — Indications for Vertebral Imaging

National Osteoporosis Foundation Recommendations for Vertebral Imaging 1

Consider vertebral imaging tests in the following individuals:

- Women ≥65 and men ≥70 years old, recommend vertebral imaging to diagnose vertebral fractures if T-score is ≤-1.5
- Women 70 and men ≥80 years old, recommend vertebral imaging to diagnose vertebral fractures, regardless of T-score
- Postmenopausal women and men ≥50 years old with a low trauma fracture
- Postmenopausal women and men age 50 to 69, recommend vertebral imaging to diagnose vertebral fractures if there is historical height loss of ≥1.5 inches, prospective height loss of ≥0.8 inches, or recent or ongoing long-term glucocorticoid treatment

International Society for Clinical Densitometry Recommendations for Vertebral Imaging 2

Lateral spine imaging by radiography or densitometric VFA is indicated when the T-score is < -1.0 and one or more of the following is present:

- Women age ≥70 years or men ≥80 years of age
- Historical height losss >4 cm (>1.5 inches)
- Self-reported but undocumented prior vertebral fracture
- Glucocorticoid therapy equivalent to ≥5 mg of prednisone or equivalent per day for ≥3 months

Modified from Cosman F, et al. *Osteoporos Int.* 2014;25:2359-2381.

REFERENCES

1. NIH Consensus Development Panel on Osteoporosis Prevention, Diagnosis, and Therapy. Osteoporosis prevention, diagnosis, and therapy. *JAMA*. 2001;285(6):785-795.

2. Assessment of fracture risk and its application to screening for postmenopausal osteoporosis. Report of a WHO Study Group. *World Health Organ Tech Rep Ser*. 1994;843:1-129.

3. Kanis JA, Melton LJ 3rd, Christiansen C, et al. The diagnosis of osteoporosis. *J Bone Miner Res*. 1994;9(8):1137-1141.

4. Baim S, Binkley N, Bilezikian JP, et al. Official Positions of the International Society for Clinical Densitometry and executive summary of the 2007 ISCD Position Development Conference. *J Clin Densitom*. 2008;11(1):75-91.

5. Official ISCD Positions Adult & Pediatric. International Society for Clinical Densitometry. https://www.iscd.org/official positions/. Last modified July 13, 2016. Accessed May 30, 2017.

6. Siris ES, Boonen S, Mitchell PJ, et al. What's in a name? What constitutes the clinical diagnosis of osteoporosis? *Osteoporos Int*. 2012;23(8):2093-2097.

7. Klotzbuecher CM, Ross PD, Landsman PB, et al. Patients with prior fractures have an increased risk of future fractures: a summary of the literature and statistical synthesis. *J Bone Miner Res*. 2000;15(4):721-739.

8. Lindsay R, Silverman SL, Cooper C, et al. Risk of new vertebral fracture in the year following a fracture. *JAMA*. 2001; 285(3):320-323.

9. Marshall D, Johnell O, Wedel H. Meta-analysis of how well measures of bone mineral density predict occurrence of osteoporotic fractures. *BMJ*. 1996;312(7041):1254-1259.

10. Mackey DC, Lui LY, Cawthon PM, et al. High-trauma fractures and low bone mineral density in older women and men. *JAMA*. 2007;298:2381-2388.

11. Harrison RA, Siminoski K, Vethanayagam D, et al. Osteoporosis-related kyphosis and impairments in pulmonary function: a systematic review. *J Bone Miner Res*. 2007;22(3):447-457.

12. Ballane G, Cauley JA, Luckey MM, El-Hajj Fuleihan G. Worldwide prevalence and incidence of osteoporotic vertebral fractures. *Osteoporos Int*. 2017;28(5):1531-1542.

13. Kiebzak GM, Beinart GA, Perser K, et al. Undertreatment of osteoporosis in men with hip fracture. *Arch Intern Med*. 2002; 162(19):2217-2222.

FIGURE 5.9 — Schematic Diagram of a Semiquantitative Grading Scale for Vertebral Fractures

0: Normal unfractured vertebra
0.5: Uncertain or questionable vertebra

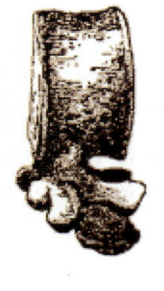

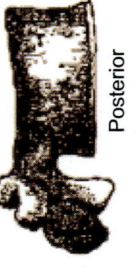

Normal/Uncertain

1: A MILD deformity with a 20% to 25% reduction in anterior, middle, and/or posterior height (relative to the same or adjacent vertebra) accompanied by a reduction in area of approximately 10% to 20%

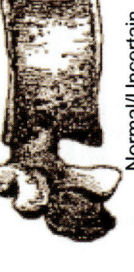

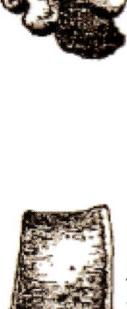

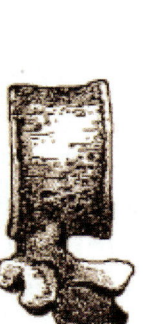

Anterior

Middle
Mild Fractures

Posterior

2: A MODERATE deformity with a >25% to 40% reduction in any height and an approximate 20% to 40% reduction in area

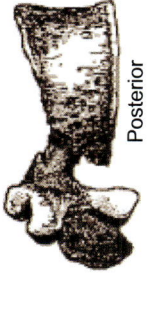

Anterior

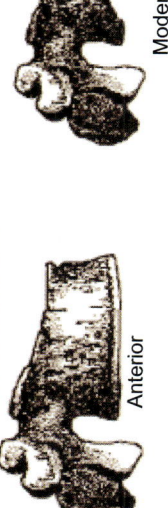

Middle
Moderate Fractures

Posterior

3: A SEVERE deformity with a >40% reduction in any height and accompanying area

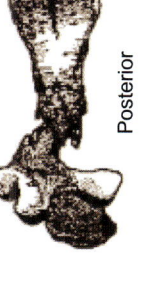

Anterior

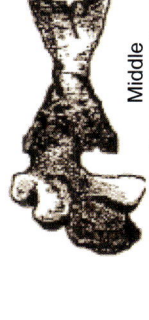

Middle
Severe Fractures

Posterior

Genant HK, Jergas M. *Osteoporos Int*. 2003;14(suppl 3):S43-S55.

FIGURE 5.10 — The Trabecular Bone Score

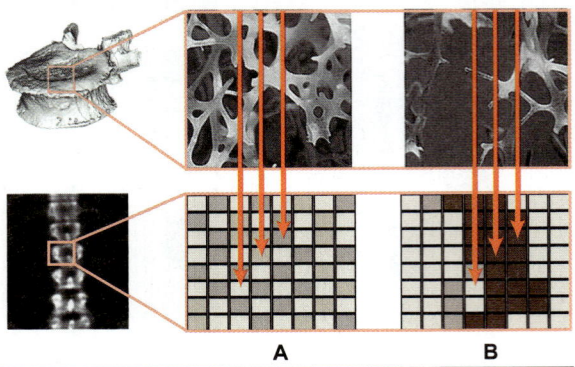

                    A   **B**

Healthy *(A)* vs altered *(B)* trabecular structures. The trabecular bone score is calculated from DXA images.

Hans D, et al. *J Clin Densitom.* 2011;14(3):302-312.

14. Valizadeh M, Mazloomzadeh S, Golmohammadi S, et al. Mortality after low trauma hip fracture: a prospective cohort study. *BMC Musculoskelet Disord.* 2012;13:143.

15. Kaukonen JP, Karaharju EO, Porras M, Lüthje P, Jakobsson A. Functional recovery after fractures of the distal forearm. Analysis of radiographic and other factors affecting the outcome. *Ann Chir Gynaecol.* 1988;77(1):27-31.

16. Cosman F, de Beur SJ, LeBoff MS, et al. Clinician's guide to prevention and treatment of osteoporosis. *Osteoporos Int.* 2014; 25:2359-2381.

17. Tannenbaum C, Clark J, Schwartzman K, et al. Yield of laboratory testing to identify secondary contributors to osteoporosis in otherwise healthy women. *J Clin Endocrinol Metab.* 2002;87(10):4431-4437.

18. Peel NF, Johnson A, Barrington NA, et al. Impact of anomalous vertebral segmentation on measurements of bone mineral density. *J Bone Miner Res.* 1993;8(6):719-723.

19. FRAX®: Fracture Risk Assessment Tool Web site. http://www.sheffield.ac.uk/FRAX/. Accessed May 30, 2017.

20. Goh JC, Low SL, Bose K. Effect of femoral rotation on bone mineral density measurements with dual energy X-ray absorptiometry. *Calcif Tissue Int.* 1995;57(5):340-343.

21. Morgan SL, Prater GL. Quality in dual-energy x-ray absorptiometry scans [published online ahead of print January 31, 2017]. *Bone*. doi: 10.1016/j.bone.2017.01.033.

22. Messina C. et al. Prevalence and type of errors in dual-energy x-ray absorptiometry. *Eur Radiol*. 2015;25:1504-1511.

23. Lewiecki EM, BinkleyN, Morgan SL. Best practices for dual-energy x-ray absorptiometry measurement and reporting: International Society for Clinical Densitometry Guidance. *J Clin Densitom*. 2016;19:127-140.

24. Camancho PM, Petak SM, Binkley N, et al. American Association of Clinical Endocrinologists and American College of Endocrinology clinical practice guidelines for the diagnosis and treatment of postmenopausal osteoporosis—2016. *Endocrine Practice*. 2016;22(9):1111-1118.

25. U.S. Preventive Services Task Force. Screening for osteoporosis: U.S. preventive services task force recommendation statement. *Ann Intern Med*. 2011;154(5):356-364.

26. Watts NB, Bilezikian JP, Camacho PM, et al. American Association of Clinical Endocrinologists Medical Guidelines for Clinical Practice for the diagnosis and treatment of postmenopausal osteoporosis. *Endocr Pract*. 2010;16(suppl 3):1-37.

27. US Preventive Services Task Force. Osteoporosis: Screening. Published January 2011. https://www.uspreventiveservicestaskforce.org/Page/Document/UpdateSummaryFinal/osteoporosis-screening. Accessed May 31, 2017.

28. National Osteoporosis Guideline Group (NOGG). Guideline for the diagnosis and management of osteoporosis in postmenopausal women and men from the age of 50 years in the UK. The University of Sheffield Web site. http://www.sheffield.ac.uk/NOGG/NOGG_Pocket_Guide_for_Healthcare_Professionals.pdf. Updated March 2014. Accessed May 30, 2017.

29. Kanis JA, McCloskey EV, Johansson H, et al. European guidance for the diagnosis and management of osteoporosis in postmenopausal women. *Osteoporos Int*. 2013;24:23-57.

30. Department of Health & Human Services (DHHS), Centers for Medicare & Medicaid Services (CMS). CMS Manual System: Pub 100-02 Medicare Benefit Policy. CMS Web site. https://www.cms.gov/Regulations-and-Guidance/Guidance/Manuals/Internet-Only-Manuals-Ioms-Items/Cms012673.html. Accessed May 30, 2017.

31. Gourlay ML, Fine JP, Preisser JS, et al. Bone-density testing interval and transition to osteoporosis in older women. *N Engl J Med*. 2012;366(3):225-233.

5

32. Gourlay ML, Overman RA, Fine JP, et al. Time to osteoporosis and major fracture in older men. The MrOS study. *Am J Prev Med*. 2016;50(6):727-736.

33. Guglielmi G, Muscarella S, Bazzocchi A. Integrated imaging approach to osteoporosis: state-of-the-art review and update. *Radiographics*. 2011;31(5):1343-1364.

34. Link TM. Osteoporosis imaging: state of the art and advanced imaging. *Radiology*. 2012;263(1):3-17.

35. Gluer CC. Quantitative ultrasound techniques for the assessment of osteoporosis: expert agreement on current status. The International Quantitative Ultrasound Consensus Group. *J Bone Miner Res*. 1997;12(8):1280-1288.

36. Guglielmi G, Scalzo G, de Terlizzi F, et al. Quantitative ultrasound in osteoporosis and bone metabolism pathologies. *Radiol Clin North Am*. 2010;48(3):577-588.

37. Naessen T, Mallmin H, Ljunghall S. Heel ultrasound in women after long-term ERT compared with bone densities in the forearm, spine and hip. *Osteoporos Int*. 1995;5(3):205-210.

38. Varenna M, Sinigaglia L, Adami S, et al. Association of quantitative heel ultrasound with history of osteoporotic fractures in elderly men: the ESOPO study. *Osteoporos Int*. 2005;16(12):1749-1754.

39. Hoiberg MP, Rubin KH, Hermann Ap, Brixen K, Abrahamsen B. Diagnostic devices for osteoporosis in the general population: a systematic review. *Bone*. 2016;92:58-69.

40. The International Society for Clinical Densitometry (ISCD), International Osteoporosis Foundation (IOF). 2010 Official Positions on FRAX®. ISCD Web site. http://www.iscd.org/wp-content/uploads/2012/10/Official-Positions-ISCD-IOF-FRAX.pdf. Published November 2010. Accessed May 30, 2017.

41. Genant HK, Jergas M. Assessment of prevalent and incident vertebral fractures in osteoporosis research. *Osteoporos Int*. 2003;14(suppl 3):S43-S55.

42. Hans D, Barthe N, Boutroy S, et al. Correlations between trabecular bone score, measured using anteroposterior dual-energy X-ray absorptiometry acquisition, and 3-dimensional parameters of bone microarchitecture: an experimental study on human cadaver vertebrae. *J Clin Densitom*. 2011;14(3):302-312.

43. Martineau P, Leslie WD. Trabecular bone score (TBS): Method and applications [published online ahead of print February 1, 2017]. *Bone*. doi: 10.1016/j.bone.2017.01.035.

44. Silva BC, Leslie WD. Trabecular Bone Score A new DXA-derived measurement for fracture risk assessment. *Endocrinol Metab Clin N Am*. 2017;46:153-180.

45. Martineau P, Leslie WD, Johansson H, et al. Clinical utility of using lumbar spine trabecular bone score to adjust fracture probability: The Manitoba Cohort [published online ahead of print March 9, 2017]. *J Bone Miner Res*. doi: 10.1002/jbmr.3124.

5

6

Diagnosis: Biochemical Markers of Bone Remodeling

Dual X-ray absorptiometry (DXA) assessment of BMD is a static indicator of bone health and does not reflect the current activity of the bone-remodeling cycle. As noted in *Chapter 2*, bone resorption is initiated by activation of osteoclasts, whose primary function is to remove old bone and to set the stage for osteoblasts to lay down osteoid, which is mineralized to form new and structurally stronger bone.

The structure and composition of bone influences the loads it can bear and, conversely, the loads that bone sustains determine its structure. The cellular process of bone modeling and remodeling mediates this adaptive mechanism. Bone remodeling prevents and repairs bone damage, thus extensive suppression of remodeling by antiresorptive agents may lead to microdamage accumulation and reduced bone strength.

Assessment of bone turnover can be achieved by measuring biochemical bone turnover markers (BTM) that fall into two categories—bone formation and bone resorption markers (**Table 6.1**).[1] The resorption of bone by osteoclasts results in the release of collagen breakdown products that can be measured in the serum and urine and comprise bone resorption markers. As bone formation occurs, osteoblasts produce type-I collagen and biochemical bone formation markers that are measurable in serum. In addition, osteoblasts secrete noncollagenous proteins that serve as markers of osteoblast activity.

Bone markers appear to be correlated with change in BMD among postmenopausal women, and high turnover is an independent risk factor for fracture.[2,3] Bone markers also have potential in monitoring the response to osteoporosis medications.[4]

TABLE 6.1 — Biochemical Bone Turnover Markers

Formation	Assay	Resorption	Assay
Total alkaline phosphatase	S	Pyridinium cross links	
Bone-specific alkaline phosphatase (BSAP)	S	Deoxypyridinoline (DPD)	U
Osteocalcin (bone GLA-protein)	S	Pyridinoline	U
Procollagen I terminal peptides		Type 1 collagen cross-linked terminal telopeptides	
Procollagen type I N-terminal peptide (P1NP)	S	N-terminal cross-linking telopeptide (NTX)	S,U
Procollagen type I C-terminal peptide (P1CP)	S	C-terminal cross-linking telopeptide (CTX)	S,U
		Tartrate-resistant acid phosphatase (TRACP5b)	S

Key: S, serum; U, urine.

Markers of Bone Formation

■ **Bone-Specific Alkaline Phosphatase**

Bone-specific alkaline phosphatase is a commonly used marker of bone formation and is reflective of osteoblast function.[5] The laboratory's reference values ensure that repeat tests use the same assay and are performed in the same laboratory. The bone-specific alkaline phosphatase isoenzyme test (using monoclonal antibodies) must be differentiated from the nonspecific total alkaline phosphatase assay routinely performed as part of liver function tests. This assay lacks sensitivity and specificity as a BTM and may be indicative of other metabolic activity or pathology affecting the liver, biliary tract, or pancreas.

■ **Osteocalcin or Bone GLA-Protein**

This protein is specific to bone and related tissues. Osteocalcin secretion is circadian, with the peak level at 4 AM and the nadir at 5 PM.[6] This cyclic activity is said to reflect an increase of bone turnover at night. The difference between peak and trough values is approximately 15%. The value of this marker as a specific indicator of osteoblast activity is confounded by its recent discovered role as a hormone that regulates pancreatic β-cell insulin secretion and insulin sensitivity.[7]

■ **Procollagen I Terminal Peptides**

Procollagen is secreted by osteoblasts and undergoes an initial proteolytic cleavage of the N- and C- terminal ends. The products, procollagen type I N-terminal peptide (P1NP) and procollagen type I C-terminal peptide (P1CP), can be detected in the serum and are useful markers of bone formation (**Figure 6.1**).

Markers of Bone Resorption

■ **Pyridinium Cross Links**

During osteoclastic bone resorption, collagen fibrils are degraded. Circulating breakdown products

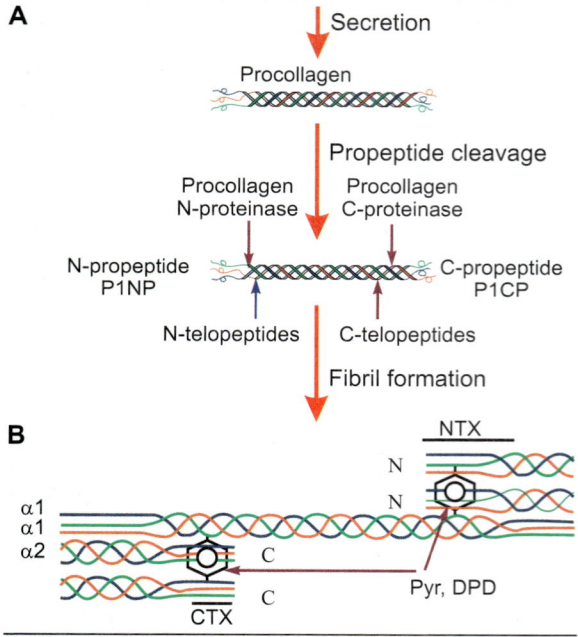

During bone formation, type I collagen molecule is synthesized as procollagen, then N-terminal and C-terminal propeptides (P1NP and P1CP, respectively) are cleaved. The central part of the molecule, triple helix of collagen, is incorporated into bone matrix *(A)*. During bone resorption, different products of the breakdown of type I collagen are produced: cross-link molecules (pyridinoline [Pyr], deoxypyridinoline [DPD]) and C-terminal and N-terminal telopeptides (CTX and NTX, respectively) *(B)*.

Modified from Szulc P, et al. *Osteoporos Int*. 2007;18:1451-1461.

as a result of this degradation serve as useful markers of bone resorption. Pyridinium cross links connect the N-terminal end of type 1 collagen molecule to the C-terminal end of an adjacent type 1 collagen molecule. The products measured are deoxypyridinoline (DPD) and pyridinoline (Pyr) (**Figure 6.1**).

■ Type 1 Collagen Cross-Linked Terminal Telopeptides

Pyridinium cross-links with fragments of collagen still attached represent other markers of bone turnover. Among these are the C-terminal (CTX) and N-terminal (NTX) cross-linking teleopeptides of the type I collagen molecule (**Figure 6.1**). They are released into the circulation and ultimately excreted in urine.

■ Tartrate-Resistant Acid Phosphatase 5b (TRACP5b)

Another marker of interest is serum tartrate-resistant acid phosphatase 5b (TRACP5b), an enzyme derived from osteoclasts. TRACP5b may reflect the number of osteoclasts, rather than their activity.

6

Bone Turnover Markers in Clinical Practice

The International Osteoporosis Foundation (IOF) and the International Federation of Clinical Chemistry and Laboratory Medicine (IFCC) recommend that the serum BTM for bone formation, P1NP, and the serum BTM for bone resorption, CTX be used as reference analytes in clinical studies.[8] Although BTMs can be measured in either blood or urine, blood is considered the preferred medium because there is significantly less intra-individual variation for blood than for urine—urine measurements must be corrected for creatinine, which adds to variation.[9] In either case, sample collection is relatively noninvasive, and the results add to the information obtained through BMD measurements. The bone resorption marker CTX is very dependent on time of day and food, and should be collected after an overnight fast.[10] Its variability is also affected by liver and renal function, and circadian rhythm.

A shortcoming of BTMs is the lack of testing standardization among laboratories and assays. Other sources of variability that has been recognized include conditions for sample collection and storage, individual patient characteristics and conditions that may acutely change BTM results such as fracture and bone metastasis. For example, the urine assays should optimally be measured on the second morning void.

■ BTMs as Predictors of Bone Fracture Risk

Changes in markers of bone formation and resorption are significantly associated with fracture risk in clinical trials and may explain more of the variance than BMD.[2,11-13] It has also been shown that an increased level of BTMs—an indicator of high bone turnover—in women with low BMD has an additive effect on risk of fracture and that the association of BTMs with fracture risk is partially independent of BMD.[14]

BTMs also may predict the rate of bone loss.[15] In concert with demographic variables, BTMs predict 30% to 40% of the variance in bone loss in untreated postmenopausal women.[14] At present, BTMs are not included in the FRAX risk assessment algorithm because of a lack of population-based prospective studies with any single BTM. One circumstance when BTMs are clinically useful in fracture risk prediction is among premenopausal women with low bone mass. Since the vast majority of these women do not have osteoporosis but more simply have low bone mass, BTM values in the premenopausal reference range provides further evidence that bone is remodeling normally and that fracture risk is likely low.[16]

■ BTMs in Monitoring Osteoporosis Therapy

In individual patients, changes in BMD as a result of osteoporosis treatment can only be reliably detected after several months (anabolic therapies) or 2 to 3 years (antiresorptive therapies), leading to a delay in the evaluation of response to treatment. In contrast, BTMs may exhibit large and rapid responses to therapy.[17,18] The reduction in marker values—those for bone resorption in particular—occurs within days or weeks after initiation of treatment with an antiresorptive agent, allowing a more rapid evaluation of therapeutic response. BTMs thus have potential in monitoring the efficacy and the adherence to therapeutic intervention. However, the biological and assay variability currently limits the utility of this approach in individual patients and requires that there be large changes between serial measurements to draw meaningful conclusions. Although variations in BTM levels as a result of treatment with both antiresorptive and anabolic therapy are associated with changes in BMD, changes in the latter do not strongly correlate to fracture risk reduction—especially for antiresorptive agents. Nevertheless, studies have shown that the larger the decrease in BTM levels, the larger the reduction in fracture risk.

When using these BTMs for treatment evaluation it is important to realize that different treatments have different cellular mechanisms of action, and BTMs need to be chosen accordingly. To use BTMs for treatment monitoring, there should be a baseline assessment with a repeat measurement at a defined interval. The detection of a difference between the chosen time points depends on drug potency, precision of measurements, and intra-individual variability. A newer potential application of BTMs is during the deliberate discontinuation of long-term bisphosphonates (a "drug holiday"). Several of the potent bisphosphonates remain within bone for months to years following therapy discontinuation leading to a protracted suppression of bone remodeling. Thus, BTMs could theoretically be useful as an indicator of when resumption of prior therapy should occur.[19,20] Studies to date have not confirmed the clinical utility of this approach.

REFERENCES

1. Calvo MS, Eyre DR, Gundberg CM. Molecular basis and clinical application of biological markers of bone turnover. *Endocr Rev.* 1996;17:333-368.

2. Garnero P, Sornay-Rendu E, Claustrat B, Delmas PD. Biochemical markers of bone turnover, endogenous hormones and the risk of fractures in postmenopausal women: the OFELY study. *J Bone Miner Res.* 2000;15:1526-1536.

3. Garnero P. Markers of bone turnover in prostate cancer. *Cancer Treat Rev.* 2001;27:187-192.

4. Greenspan SL, Resnick NM, Parker RA. Early changes in biochemical markers of bone turnover are associated with long-term changes in bone mineral density in elderly women on alendronate, hormone replacement therapy, or combination therapy: a three-year, double-blind, placebo-controlled, randomized clinical trial. *J Clin Endocrinol Metab.* 2005;90:2762-2767.

5. Gomez B Jr, Ardakani S, Ju J, et al. Monoclonal antibody assay for measuring bone-specific alkaline phosphatase activity in serum. *Clin Chem.* 1995;41:1560-1566.

6. Markowitz ME, Gundberg CM, Rosen JF. The circadian rhythm of serum osteocalcin concentrations: effects of 1,25 dihydroxyvitamin D administration. *Calcif Tissue Int.* 1987;40:179-183.

7. Ferron M, Wei J, Yoshizawa T, et al. Insulin signaling in osteoblasts integrates bone remodeling and energy metabolism. *Cell.* 2010;142:296-308.

8. Vasikaran S, Eastell R, Bruyere O, et al. Markers of bone turnover for the prediction of fracture risk and monitoring of osteoporosis treatment: a need for international reference standards. *Osteoporos Int.* 2011;22:391-420.

9. Hannon R, Eastell R. Preanalytical variability of biochemical markers of bone turnover. *Osteoporos Int.* 2000;11(suppl 6):S30-S44.

10. Qvist P, Christgau S, Pedersen BJ, Schlemmer A, Christiansen C. Circadian variation in the serum concentration of C-terminal telopeptide of type I collagen (serum CTx): effects of gender, age, menopausal status, posture, daylight, serum cortisol, and fasting. *Bone.* 2002;31:57-61.

11. Garnero P, Sornay-Rendu E, Chapuy MC, Delmas PD. Increased bone turnover in late postmenopausal women is a major determinant of osteoporosis. *J Bone Miner Res.* 1996;11:337-349.

12. Ivaska KK, Gerdhem P, Vaananen HK, Akesson K, Obrant KJ. Bone turnover markers and prediction of fracture: a prospective follow-up study of 1040 elderly women for a mean of 9 years. *J Bone Miner Res*. 2010;25:393-403.

13. Sornay-Rendu E, Munoz F, Garnero P, Duboeuf F, Delmas PD. Identification of osteopenic women at high risk of fracture: the OFELY study. *J Bone Miner Res.* 2005;20:1813-1819.

14. Johnell O, Oden A, De Laet C, Garnero P, Delmas PD, Kanis JA. Biochemical indices of bone turnover and the assessment of fracture probability. *Osteoporos Int*. 2002;13:523-526.

15. Rogers A, Hannon RA, Eastell R. Biochemical markers as predictors of rates of bone loss after menopause. *J Bone Miner Res*. 2000;15:1398-1404.

16. de Papp AE, Bone HG, Caulfield MP, et al. A cross-sectional study of bone turnover markers in healthy premenopausal women. *Bone*. 2007;40:1222-1230.

17. Bauer DC, Black DM, Garnero P, et al. Change in bone turnover and hip, non-spine, and vertebral fracture in alendronate-treated women: the fracture intervention trial. *J Bone Miner Res.* 2004;19:1250-1258.

18. Chen P, Satterwhite JH, Licata AA, et al. Early changes in biochemical markers of bone formation predict BMD response to teriparatide in postmenopausal women with osteoporosis. *J Bone Miner Res*. 2005;20:962-970.

19. Ravn P, Christensen JO, Baumann M, Clemmesen B. Changes in biochemical markers and bone mass after withdrawal of ibandronate treatment: prediction of bone mass changes during treatment. *Bone*. 1998;22:559-564.

20. Black DM, Schwartz AV, Ensrud KE, et al. Effects of continuing or stopping alendronate after 5 years of treatment: the Fracture Intervention Trial Long-term Extension (FLEX): a randomized trial. *JAMA*. 2006;296:2927-2938.

6

7

Prevention and Treatment: Nonpharmacologic Therapy

Countless thousands of women following vertebral fractures experience physical and psychological chronic pain. In addition to prescription and nonprescription drugs, as well as calcium and vitamins, much can be done to treat this pain, prevent fractures, and improve the quality of life of women through nondrug means. Approaches to nonpharmacologic therapy for osteoporosis prevention and treatment include:

- General exercise and physical therapy
- Fall prevention programs
- Mechanical hip protectors
- Vertebroplasty and kyphoplasty.

General Exercise and Physical Therapy

Exercise assumes an important role in achieving optimal peak bone mass, but data regarding its effects on prevention of fracture—which is the principal goal of physical exercise in those at risk for fracture—are limited. In young healthy adults, it has been established that any physical activity can be important in achieving a greater peak bone mass, bone strength, and geometry. Achieving optimal BMD before menopause is a major factor in reducing the risk of fracture. Among premenopausal women, programs that combine high-impact exercise with high-magnitude exercise in the form of resistance training including rope jumping, running, aerobics, bounding exercises, and unaccustomed movements effectively increase BMD at the lumbar spine as well as the femoral neck.[1] The bone area receiving the bulk of the biomechanical loading typically experiences the greatest increase in BMD. For example,

BMD proportionately increases most in the dominant arm of racquet sport players. Moreover, a number of studies have demonstrated that exercise prescriptions can maintain or increase BMD in postmenopausal women as well. In that population, aerobics, weight-bearing exercise, and resistance exercise were effective in enhancing spine BMD.[2] Notably, walking programs showed no significant effect on spine BMD but were effective at the hip. For subjects with increased fracture risk—low BMD or osteoporosis—bone strength appears to be improved through weight-bearing aerobic exercise with or without muscle-strengthening exercise, if subjects engaged in the program for at least a year.

It should be noted, however, that the benefits gained through exercise on muscle power, muscle strength, body balance, gait, BMD, or number of falls does not necessarily result in a reduction of fractures. For example, although BMD loss over time at the hip is associated with an increased fracture risk, the converse is not inevitable; an exercise-induced increase in BMD has not been shown to be associated with a reduction in fracture incidence.

There is some indirect evidence that encourages the use of exercise interventions to reduce fracture risk. It is generally recommended that patients be engaged in exercise programs two to three times per week, with a goal of 15 to 60 minutes of aerobic activity, at an intensity of 70% to 80% of functional capacity. High impact exercise should be included where possible since it has the greatest effect on improving BMD.[3] Because high impact exercise may not be appropriate for those not used to exercising, for those over age 50, or for those with significant existing deficits in bone mass, low to medium impact exercise, such as brisk walking, step aerobics, or intermittent jogging, can be advised.

In addition, for those with osteoporosis, strength training should be site specific, focusing on muscle groups surrounding the hips, for example, as well as the quadriceps, dorsi/plantar flexors, wrist extensors, and back extensors. Weight-bearing exercise should pinpoint loading bone sites most likely to be affected by fracture risk. In addition, adding weight-bearing and resistance exercise to a routine medication regimen provided greater improvements in BMD than either physical exercise or medication alone.

An osteoporosis exercise program is often best devised by a physical therapist. In addition to instructing in a particular exercise program, physical therapy should also focus on the maintaining a healthy spinal alignment aimed at avoiding spinal fractures and reducing back pain that may result from osteoporotic fractures or associated postural changes, faulty body mechanics, and weak back musculature. Avoidance of excessive spine flexion and rotation may also prevent vertebral fractures.

Physical therapy approaches for improving back pain due to osteoporosis associated thoracic kyphosis:

- Correct posture
- Develop good body mechanics
- Strengthen back and stabilization muscles.

All of the above issues are exaggerated by the physical deformity and associated muscle pain that occurs with vertebral fractures.

Therapeutic protocols include:

- Mental imagery:
  - Dropping an imaginary plumb line from head to toe
  - Think tall
  - Maintain a level pelvis
  - Lengthen the midsection of the body
- Site-specific exercises to strengthen regional muscle groups
- Balance: evaluation and correction of problems with:
  - Vision
  - Hearing
  - Muscle strength
  - Posture
  - Relationship between the following:

- Feet on the ground
- Movement
- Awareness of head position
- Walking: misalignment of the hip may be a significant contributor to low back pain
- Scapular stabilization: strengthening the scapular muscles is important for posture and relief of the frequently complained of "burning" back pain
- Activities of daily living, which include everyday activities and ways of ensuring that incorrect body mechanics do not aggravate the underlying pathology. Guidance is given for how best to deal with:
  - Standing
  - Sitting
  - Lifting and carrying
  - Daily activities in the bedroom, bathroom, and kitchen
  - Housework
  - Yardwork
  - Driving a car
  - Pet care.

The importance of attention to activities of daily living by a physical therapist, occupational therapist, or other health care provider, will aid the rehabilitation of patients with osteoporosis.

Fall Prevention

Among community-dwelling adults >65 years of age, between 28% and 35% experience at least one fall each year, and the annual fall prevalence increases with aging.[4,5] Between 10% and 31% are recurrent fallers.[6] Progressive balance, gait, and strength training, as well as Tai Chi, are effective for fall prevention.[7-10] One meta-analysis of muscle-strengthening and balance-retraining exercise programs for men and women aged 65 to 97 years showed a reduction in falls and fall-related injuries of 35%.

A short, multidisciplinary falls-prevention program in women with osteoporosis and a fall history can lower falls by nearly 40% and significantly increase balance but may not affect quality of life (QOL) or activity levels.[11] A 12-month balance-training program involving elderly osteoporotic women led to significant improvement in balance and functional mobility, as well as a greater reduction in the number of falls in the intervention group.[12]

Balance and strength programs carefully designed for elderly patients—including those with osteoporosis—can reduce the risk of falls and the inherent danger of fractures.

Mechanical Hip Protectors

As illustrated in **Figure 3.3**, women who fracture their hip do so because they have lost both their sense of balance and protective reflex mechanism through loss of muscle strength and other factors. Instead of falling onto an outstretched arm (which usually results in a wrist fracture), they fall onto the greater trochanter of the hip. Other factors that contribute to the fracture include:

- Hip bone strength with BMD, an important surrogate marker
- The mechanical stress and force of the fall
- The soft tissue energy absorption of the fall.

Mechanical hip protectors may help to decrease the magnitude of the impact, and in one study, reduced the percent of fractures from falls by 85% (**Figure 7.1**).[13] Nevertheless, patient adherence to hip protectors is low.[14] Further, not all studies have confirmed the efficacy of hip protectors.[15] Because design and wearing comfort of hip protectors are also important factors in adherence, hip protectors with a more patient-friendly design that are incorporated in shorts or sweat pants are available.

FIGURE 7.1 — Hip Protectors Attenuate Fracture Risk

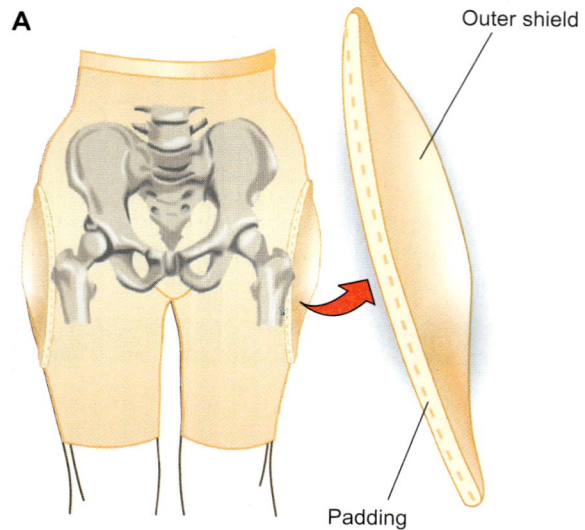

Hip fractures are caused by a fall on the greater trochanter, and the components of the fracture include the fall, hip bone strength, energy absorption, and a protective reflex mechanism; often a wrist fracture may occur in trying to protect from a fall. Hip protectors are an extrinsic device that can decrease the magnitude of the impact *(A)*. They are indicated for specific patients, ie, those who fall easily, lean people, and those with previous fractures. Other patients also may be candidates for this type of treatment.

Continued

Vertebral Stabilization

Two procedures, vertebroplasty and kyphoplasty, have been developed aimed at the relief of pain associated with vertebral compression fractures. When successful, pain relief occurs within 24 to 48 hours

Vertebroplasty is a minimally invasive technique and typically involves the placement of bone cement

FIGURE 7.1 — *Continued*

B

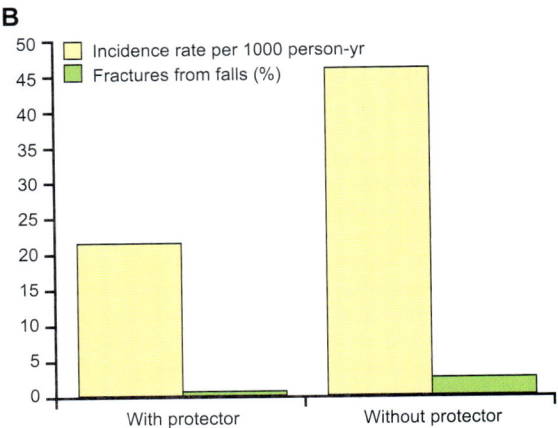

The number of hip fractures is halved when patients wear hip protectors (from 46.0 to 21.3 fractures per 1000 person-years) *(B)*. Similarly, the percent of fractures from falls is reduced by 85%, from 2.43 to 0.39 fractures per 100 falls.

Kannus P, et al. *N Engl J Med*. 2000;343:1506-1513.

(polymethylmethacrylate) directly into the fractured vertebra, thus stabilizing the fracture (**Figure 7.2**).

Kyphoplasty involves the insertion of inflatable balloons into the fractured vertebrae, elevating the end plates, and typically injecting a bone cement into the decompressed area while removing the balloon (**Figure 7.3**). This technique involves general anesthesia. It is aimed at both restoration of vertebral height and stabilization of the fracture. In some series, pain relief has been achieved in 90% of treated patients.[16-18]

Both procedures have provided significant pain relief in some but not in all studies, diminishing the requirement for analgesia.[19-22] The incidence of complications and potential problems with vertebroplasty and kyphoplasty should be discussed with patients before the procedure. Complications can include the extravasation of bone cement into the epidural space

FIGURE 7.2 — Vertebroplasty: Vertebral Compression Fracture Treatment Options

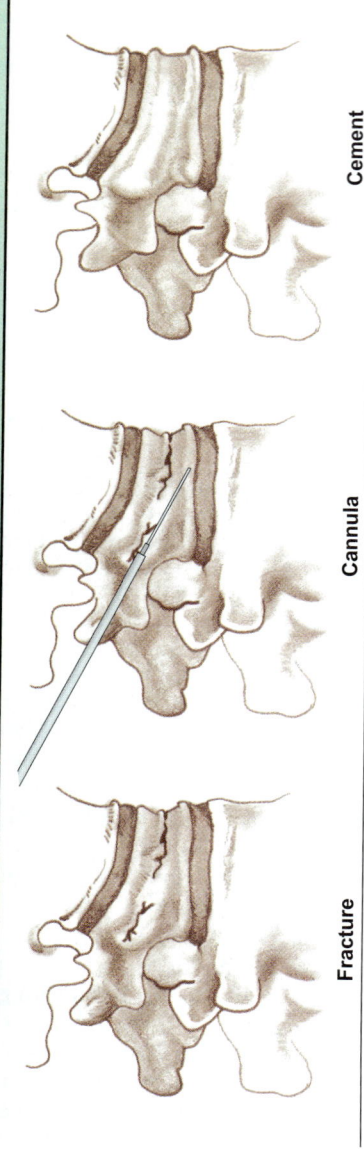

| Fracture | Cannula | Cement |

Vertebroplasty is a minimally invasive technique to introduce cement directly into a fractured vertebra, thus stabilizing the fracture. A cannula is introduced into the vertebral body from a transpedicular approach, and rather liquid cement is introduced into the fractured vertebra.

FIGURE 7.3 — Kyphoplasty for Vertebral Compression

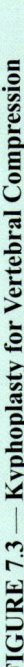

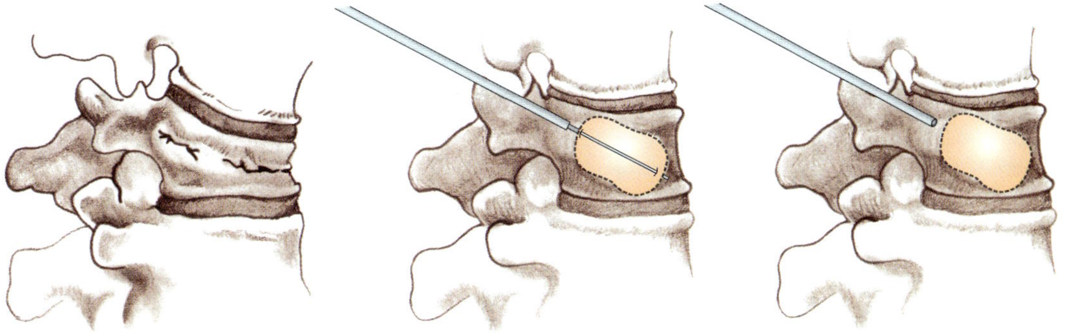

Fracture **Tamp Reduction** **Cement**

Kyphoplasty elevates the end plates of the fractured vertebra in an effort to restore vertebral height in addition to providing pain relief and fracture stabilization. The bone tamp is inserted through a working cannula from a transpedicular approach, the fracture is reduced, and then cement is introduced in a viscous state.

leading to neurologic compromise as well as immediate and delayed fractures at contiguous vertebral levels.[18]

Surgical Interventions

Surgical treatment of the osteoporotic spine is among the most challenging interventions in spinal surgery. The indications for surgical intervention for osteoporotic compression fractures have not been strictly defined. The vast majority of spinal fragility fractures occurring with low impact injuries do not lead to neurologic compromise and do not require surgical intervention. Currently, the consensus includes progressive neurological loss, severe unrelenting pain, and significant deformity. Appropriate patients have traditionally been treated with anterior decompression either through a thoracotomy or retroperitoneal approach and reconstruction of the involved level using a structural graft. However, reliable fixation may be difficult to achieve, and structural grafts frequently subside in weak osteoporotic bone. Preoperative health status must be carefully considered.

REFERENCES

1. Martyn-St James M, Carroll S. Effects of different impact exercise modalities on bone mineral density in premenopausal women: a meta-analysis. *J Bone Miner Metab*. 2010;28(3):251-267.

2. Howe TE, Shea B, Dawson LJ, et al. Exercise for preventing and treating osteoporosis in postmenopausal women. *Cochrane Database Syst Rev*. 2011;(7):CD000333.

3. Babatunde OO, Forsyth JJ, Gidlow CJ. A meta-analysis of brief high-impact exercises for enhancing bone health in premenopausal women. *Osteoporos Int*. 2012;23(1):109-119.

4. Masud T, Morris RO. Epidemiology of falls. *Age Ageing*. 2001;30(suppl 4):3-7.

5. Pluijm SM, Smit JH, Tromp EA, et al. A risk profile for identifying community-dwelling elderly with a high risk of recurrent falling: results of a 3-year prospective study. *Osteoporos Int*. 2006;17(3):417-425.

6. Body JJ, Bergmann P, Boonen S, et al. Non-pharmacological management of osteoporosis: a consensus of the Belgian Bone Club. *Osteoporos Int*. 2011;22(11):2769-2788.

7. American College of Sports Medicine, Chodzko-Zajko WJ, Proctor DN, et al. American College of Sports Medicine position stand. Exercise and physical activity for older adults. *Med Sci Sports Exerc*. 2009;41(7):1510-1530.

8. Gillespie LD, Robertson MC, Gillespie WJ, et al. Interventions for preventing falls in older people living in the community. *Cochrane Database Syst Rev*. 2012;9:CD007146.

9. Chang JT, Morton SC, Rubenstein LZ, et al. Interventions for the prevention of falls in older adults: systematic review and meta-analysis of randomised clinical trials. *BMJ*. 2004; 328(7441):680.

10. Tinetti ME, Kumar C. The patient who falls: "It's always a trade-off". *JAMA*. 2010;303(3):258-266.

11. Smulders E, Weerdesteyn V, Groen BE, et al. Efficacy of a short multidisciplinary falls prevention program for elderly persons with osteoporosis and a fall history: a randomized controlled trial. *Arch Phys Med Rehabil*. 2010;91(11):1705-1711.

12. Madureira MM, Takayama L, Gallinaro AL, Caparbo VF, Costa RA, Pereira RM. Balance training program is highly effective in improving functional status and reducing the risk of falls in elderly women with osteoporosis: a randomized controlled trial. *Osteoporos Int*. 2007;18(4):419-425.

7

13. Kannus P, Parkkari J, Niemi S, et al. Prevention of hip fracture in elderly people with use of a hip protector. *N Engl J Med.* 2000;343(21):1506-1513.

14. Holzer G, Holzer LA. Hip protectors and prevention of hip fractures in older persons. *Geriatrics.* 2007;62(8):15-20.

15. Kiel DP, Magaziner J, Zimmerman S, et al. Efficacy of a hip protector to prevent hip fracture in nursing home residents: the HIP PRO randomized controlled trial. *JAMA.* 2007;298(4):413-422.

16. Feltes C, Fountas KN, Machinis T, et al. Immediate and early postoperative pain relief after kyphoplasty without significant restoration of vertebral body height in acute osteoporotic vertebral fractures. *Neurosurg Focus.* 2005;18(3):e5.

17. Grohs JG, Matzner M, Trieb K, Krepler P. Minimal invasive stabilization of osteoporotic vertebral fractures: a prospective nonrandomized comparison of vertebroplasty and balloon kyphoplasty. *J Spinal Disord Tech.* 2005;18(3):238-242.

18. Garfin SR, Yuan HA, Reiley MA. New technologies in spine: kyphoplasty and vertebroplasty for the treatment of painful osteoporotic compression fractures. *Spine (Phila Pa 1976).* 2001;26(14):1511-1515.

19. Buchbinder R, Osborne RH, Ebeling PR, et al. A randomized trial of vertebroplasty for painful osteoporotic vertebral fractures. *N Engl J Med.* 2009;361(6):557-568.

20. Kallmes DF, Comstock BA, Heagerty PJ, et al. A randomized trial of vertebroplasty for osteoporotic spinal fractures. *N Engl J Med.* 2009;361(6):569-579.

21. Klazen CA, Lohle PN, de Vries J, et al. Vertebroplasty versus conservative treatment in acute osteoporotic vertebral compression fractures (Vertos II): an open-label randomised trial. *Lancet.* 2010;376(9746):1085-1092.

22. Wardlaw D, Cummings SR, Van Meirhaeghe J, et al. Efficacy and safety of balloon kyphoplasty compared with non-surgical care for vertebral compression fracture (FREE): a randomised controlled trial. *Lancet.* 2009;373(9668):1016-1024.

8
Prevention and Treatment: Calcium and Vitamin D

An adequate intake of various dietary components, which serve as building blocks, is important for optimal bone health. This chapter will focus on the roles of calcium and vitamin D in bone health. However, other nutrients such as protein and other vitamins and minerals are also important in bone health.

Calcium

Approximately one third of the volume and two thirds of the weight of bone is made of mineral, hydroxyapatite. Hydroxyapatite crystals in the mineralized bone contain significant amounts of sodium, magnesium, carbonate, and citrate ions, but calcium and phosphorus are the principal constituents. Calcium is approximately 40% of hydroxyapatite and 99% of the body's calcium is found in the skeleton.

Table 8.1 shows the Dietary Reference Intakes for calcium.[1,2] The higher calcium requirement for postmenopausal women is due to a combination of less efficient calcium absorption from the gut and poorer calcium reabsorption by the kidneys.

Excellent dietary sources of calcium ($\geq$200 mg/serving) include milk, yogurt, fortified fruit juices, and natural cheeses. Other good sources ($\geq$100 mg/serving) include calcium-set tofu, processed cheese, and fortified cereals. Other foods such as salmon with the bones, collards, turnip greens, and kale generally have <100 mg/serving. Not all calcium-containing foods are bioavailable; for example, the majority of the calcium in spinach is bound by oxalate. A dietary calcium calculator is available at http://www.uab.edu/shp/toneyourbones/ and is shown in **Figure 8.1**.[3]

TABLE 8.1 — Dietary Reference Intakes for Calcium and Vitamin D

Life Stage Group	Calcium			Vitamin D		
	Estimated Average Requirement (mg/day)	Recommended Dietary Allowance (mg/day)	Upper Level Intake (mg/day)	Estimated Average Requirement (IU/day)	Recommended Dietary Allowance (IU/day)	Upper Level Intake (IU/day)
Infants 0-6 months	a	a	1000	b	b	1000
Infants 6-12 months	a	a	1500	b	b	1500
1-3 years old	500	700	2500	400	600	2500
4-8 years old	800	1000	2500	400	600	3000
9-13 years old	1100	1300	3000	400	600	4000
14-18 years old	1100	1300	3000	400	600	4000
19-30 years old	800	1000	2500	400	600	4000
31-50 years old	800	1000	2500	400	600	4000
51-70 year old males	800	1000	2000	400	600	4000
51-70 year old females	1000	1200	2000	400	600	4000
>70 years old	1000	1200	2000	400	800	4000

14-18 years old, pregnant/lactating	1100	1300	3000	400	600	4000
19-50 years old, pregnant/lactating	800	1000	2500	400	600	4000

[a] For infants, adequate intake is 200 mg/day for 0 to 6 months of age and 260 mg/day for 6 to 12 months of age.
[b] For infants, adequate intake is 400 IU/day for 0 to 6 months of age and 400 IU/day for 6 to 12 months of age.

DRIs for Calcium and Vitamin D. Institute of Medicine of the National Academies Web site. http://www.iom.edu/Reports/2010/Dietary -Reference-Intakes-for-Calcium-and-Vitamin-D/DRI-Values.aspx. Released November 30, 2010. Accessed May 25, 2017.

FIGURE 8.1 — Calcium Calculator

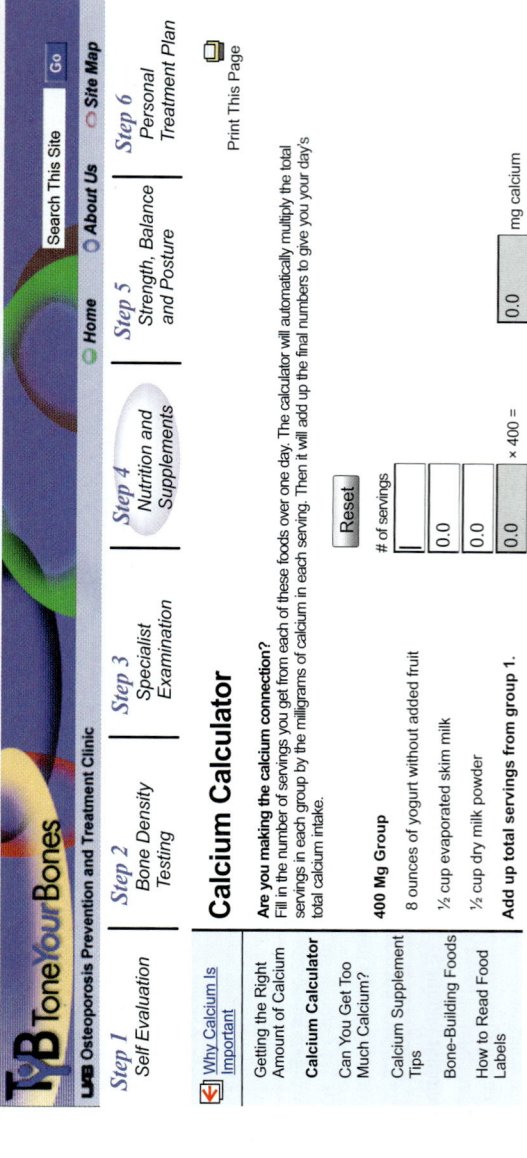

TYB ToneYour Bones

LAB Osteoporosis Prevention and Treatment Clinic

○ Home   ○ About Us   ○ Site Map

Search This Site [   ] [Go]

| *Step 1* Self Evaluation | *Step 2* Bone Density Testing | *Step 3* Specialist Examination | *Step 4* Nutrition and Supplements | *Step 5* Strength, Balance and Posture | *Step 6* Personal Treatment Plan |

🖶 Print This Page

▼ Why Calcium Is Important

Getting the Right Amount of Calcium

Calcium Calculator

Can You Get Too Much Calcium?

Calcium Supplement Tips

Bone-Building Foods

How to Read Food Labels

Calcium Calculator

Are you making the calcium connection?
Fill in the number of servings you get from each of these foods over one day. The calculator will automatically multiply the total servings in each group by the milligrams of calcium in each serving. Then it will add up the final numbers to give you your day's total calcium intake.

[Reset]

# of servings

400 Mg Group

8 ounces of yogurt without added fruit   [   ]

½ cup evaporated skim milk   [0.0]

½ cup dry milk powder   [0.0]

Add up total servings from group 1.   [0.0] × 400 =   [0.0] mg calcium

152

300 Mg Group

	# of servings
8 ounces of milk (any kind)	0.0
8 ounces of fruited yogurt	0.0
8 ounces of calcium-fortified orange juice	0.0
¼ cup parmesan cheese	0.0
½ cup part-skim ricotta cheese	0.0
1 ounce Swiss or Gruyere cheese	0.0
½ cup calcium-treated tofu	0.0
3 ounces canned sardines w/bones	0.0
Add up total servings from group 2.	0.0 × 300 =

0.0 mg calcium

200 Mg Group

	# of servings
1 ounce natural cheese	0.0
Add up total servings from group 3.	0.0 × 200 =

0.0 mg calcium

8

Continued

FIGURE 8.1 — *Continued*

150 Mg Group

	# of servings
1 packet of instant oatmeal	0.0
½ cup pudding, custard, flan	0.0
½ cup cooked collards	0.0
3 ounces pink canned salmon w/bones	0.0
Add up total servings from group 4.	0.0

0.0 × 150 = [0.0] mg calcium

100 Mg Group

	# of servings
1 ounce nonfat cream cheese	0.0
½ cup turnip greens, bok choy	0.0
1 ounce almonds	0.0
½ cup cottage cheese	0.0
½ cup ice cream, ice milk, frozen yogurt	0.0
½ cup white beans	0.0
1 serving of most calcium-fortified cereals	0.0
Add up total servings from group 5.	0.0

0.0 × 100 = [0.0] mg calcium

50 Mg Group

	# of servings
½ cup broccoli	0.0
½ cup kale, mustard greens	0.0
½ cup most dried beans	0.0
1 medium corn tortilla	0.0
1 medium orange	0.0
1 tablespoon dry milk	0.0
Add up total servings from group 6.	0.0 × 50 =

0.0 mg calcium

Now add up your total mg of calcium from each group for your day's total.

0.0

Add in calcium from supplements and compare your total to your recommended intake.

0.0

TOTAL 0.0

Reset

8

Calcium Calculator. Tone Your Bones Web site. http://www.uab.edu/shp/toneyourbones/calcium-calculator. Accessed May 25, 2017.

Figure 8.2 shows a food label. Since the reference value for calcium is based upon 1000 mg of calcium per day, if a zero is added to the % daily value for calcium on the label, it will yield the mg of calcium per serving.

- ■ **Calcium Absorption**
  - • Calcium is absorbed primarily in the proximal small intestine; maximally in the duodenum and proximal jejunum. This explains why individuals having a roux-en-y gastric bypass have problems with calcium absorption since these portions of intestine are bypassed.
  - • Absorption of calcium is complete within 4 hours of its intake and is more efficient with lower amounts of calcium.
  - • Although 75% of ingested calcium may be absorbed by children during periods of rapid skeletal growth and remodeling, the value decreases to 30% to 50% in adults.
  - • Intestinal fractional calcium absorption decreases even more in elderly women (>70 years).
  - • Calcium is needed consistently on a daily basis and lifetime intake of calcium is important. Individuals must be given the option of achieving their recommended amounts by whatever means are convenient, acceptable, and affordable.
  - • Vitamin D adequacy is essential for calcium absorption. Therefore, it is difficult to study calcium in isolation in clinical trials.

- ■ **Mean Dietary Calcium Intakes in the United States**

  Using data from the National Health and Nutrition Examination Survey (NHANES) from 2003 through 2006, it was determined that dietary intakes for most Americans do not reach the Dietary Reference Intake amounts.[4] Because dietary intakes tend to be inadequate, the use of calcium supplements is often recommended for many individuals with metabolic

FIGURE 8.2 — Interpretation of Food Labels for Calcium and Vitamin D Content

Skim Milk
Serving Size 8 fl oz (240mL)
Servings Per Container 2

Amount Per Serving

Calories 80   Calories from Fat 0

% Daily Value*

Total Fat 0g	0%
Saturated Fat 0g	0%
Cholesterol less than 5mg	1%
Sodium 130mg	5%
Total Carbohydrate 12g	4%
Dietary Fiber 0g	0%
Sugars 11g	
Protein 8g	

Vitamin A 8%   •   Vitamin C 4%

Calcium 30% • Iron 0% • Vitamin D 25%

* Percent Daily Values are based on a 2,000 calorie diet. Your daily values may be higher or lower depending on your calorie needs.

Add a zero to the % calcium daily value *(yellow highlight)*. In this instance, the amount of calcium per 8 fluid ounce serving is 300 mg. The % daily value for vitamin D is based on 400 IU. Therefore in this instance, the amount of vitamin D in 8 fluid ounces is 100 IU *(green highlight)*.

How to Read Food Labels. Tone Your Bones Website. http://www.uab.edu/shp/toneyourbones/step-4-nutrition-and-supplements/why-calcium-is-important/how-to-read-food-labels. Accessed May 25, 2017.

bone disease. The NHANES survey also demonstrated that a large proportion of men and women in the United States are using calcium supplements.[4]

■ Calcium Supplementation

Much has been written about the preferred or best type of calcium supplement. The fewer the tablets and the less expensive, the more likely it is that individuals will take supplements.

- Only elemental calcium is available for absorption. Calcium carbonate contains 40% of elemental calcium; tribasic calcium phosphate, 39%; calcium citrate, 24%; calcium lactate, 13%; and, calcium gluconate, 9%. In clinical terms, the availability of calcium from these sources does not differ significantly, however, if there is achlorhydria, calcium citrate may be used, or calcium carbonate should be taken with meals.

- It is generally recommended that an individual consume no more than 500 mg to 600 mg of calcium at a time. Calcium taken several times a day with meals is less likely to saturate the intestinal absorptive mechanism.

- A variety of calcium-fortified beverages are available. It is important to shake the calcium-fortified soy beverages before use since the fortified calcium may settle to the bottom of the container.[5] Mineral waters tend to have a calcium absorbability equivalent to milk and may be used as a way to supplement calcium intake.[6]

■ Protective Effects of Calcium on Bone

Can calcium by itself prevent osteoporosis? Although calcium supplementation in postmenopausal women has been shown to reduce or prevent bone loss, robust evidence for protection against fracture is lacking. However, when combined calcium and vitamin D supplements are used, there is reasonable evidence for small reductions in hip and nonvertebral fracture rates.[7] **Figure 8.3** reviews these data.

FIGURE 8.3 — Vitamin D and Calcium Reduce Fracture Risk

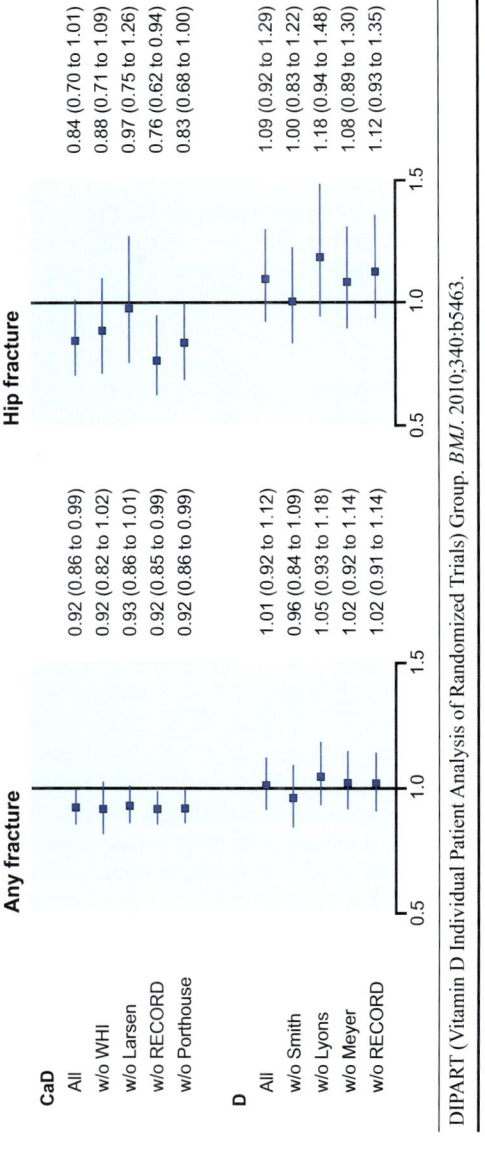

Any fracture

Hip fracture

CaD

	Any fracture	Hip fracture
All	0.92 (0.86 to 0.99)	0.84 (0.70 to 1.01)
w/o WHI	0.92 (0.82 to 1.02)	0.88 (0.71 to 1.09)
w/o Larsen	0.93 (0.86 to 1.01)	0.97 (0.75 to 1.26)
w/o RECORD	0.92 (0.85 to 0.99)	0.76 (0.62 to 0.94)
w/o Porthouse	0.92 (0.86 to 0.99)	0.83 (0.68 to 1.00)

D

	Any fracture	Hip fracture
All	1.01 (0.92 to 1.12)	1.09 (0.92 to 1.29)
w/o Smith	0.96 (0.84 to 1.09)	1.00 (0.83 to 1.22)
w/o Lyons	1.05 (0.93 to 1.18)	1.18 (0.94 to 1.48)
w/o Meyer	1.02 (0.92 to 1.14)	1.08 (0.89 to 1.30)
w/o RECORD	1.02 (0.91 to 1.14)	1.12 (0.93 to 1.35)

DIPART (Vitamin D Individual Patient Analysis of Randomized Trials) Group. *BMJ.* 2010;340:b5463.

A 2013 report from the US Preventive Services Task Force recommended against the use of 1000 mg of calcium (with 400 IU of vitamin D or less) for the primary prevention of fractures in non-institutionalized older adults.[8] It should be noted that this recommendation does not apply to persons with osteoporosis and it addresses only supplements, not total daily calcium intake.

In nearly all of the clinical trials of pharmacologic interventions for osteoporosis, calcium and vitamin D supplements have been given as an adjunct to treatment. Calcium supplements should therefore be considered in such patients if dietary intake is inadequate.

A review of milk and dairy products related to health found that such products have a beneficial effect on bone density but no effect on fractures. Milk and dairy products improve body composition and facilitate weight loss and their intake is neutral or confers a reduced risk of type 2 diabetes and confer a reduced risk of cardiovascular disease/stroke.[9]

■ Side Effects of Calcium Supplementation

The tolerability of calcium supplements may be poor and therefore adherence correspondingly low in some individuals. Gastrointestinal symptoms are a common reason for stopping therapy and when they occur, switching to alternative formulations/calcium salts should be considered. Calcium supplements now come in a broad array of forms and sizes (pills, chews, liquids, and crystals that dissolve in water). If there is constipation, a calcium supplement containing magnesium may be used, if there is no contraindication to magnesium supplementation.

There has been controversy about whether calcium supplementation increases the risk of cardiovascular events, with analysis suggesting that calcium supplements are detrimental to cardiovascular health.[10-12] The Heidelberg cohort was an observational cohort study investigating the effect of dietary and calcium supplements on stroke, myocardial infarction, and cardiovascular mortality.[13] In their study, calcium supplement users have a statistically significant increase in myocardial infarction risk compared to nonusers of supplements; however, there was no increase in stroke risk or cardiovascular mortality.

In an analysis of data from the Women's Health Trial, calcium and vitamin D supplementation did not increase the risk of myocardial infarction, coronary heart disease, total heart disease, stroke, or overall cardiovascular disease.[14] An analysis of calcium supplement use from the Nurse's Health Study did not find that the use of calcium supplements increased CVD risk in women.[15]

Calcium intake has not been associated with increased coronary artery calcification in analysis from the Framingham Study[16] and also was not associated with increased carotid artery intimal thickness or atherosclerosis.[17] In thinking about the mechanism of atherosclerotic plaque formation, it is clear that calcification of vessels is a response and is not a cause of atherosclerosis.[18]

A meta-analysis of clinical trials, using verified coronary artery disease, myocardial infarction, angina pectoris, acute coronary syndrome, and coronary heart disease in individuals taking calcium supplements vs placebo did not find that calcium supplements, with or without vitamin D, increased coronary heart disease or all-cause mortality in elderly women.[19] A meta-analysis of studies from 1966 to July 2016 of randomized trials, prospective cohort and nested case-control studied with data on calcium supplements (with or without vitamin D) and cardiovascular outcomes concluded that calcium intake within 2000-2500 mg/day is not associated with increase cardiovascular disease risk in healthy adults.[20]

A clinical guideline from the National Osteoporosis Foundation and the American Society for Preventive Cardiology has concluded that in generally healthy adults when calcium intake from food and supplements does not exceed 2000-2500 mg/day, that there is neither benefit nor risk related to cardiovascular and cerebrovascular disease mortality, or all-cause mortality.[21] In counseling patients related to calcium intake, it is reasonable to first maximize calcium intake from dietary sources and then fill in with supplements as necessary to achieve a goal intake.

A potential side effect of calcium supplementation is the development of renal stones, which was seen in the WHI Trial.[22] The bone physiology of renal stone formers is different than in individuals with hypercalciuria who do not form renal stones, with stone formers typically having lower BMD than individuals with hypercalciuria and no stones.[23,24] Studies of individuals who have had calcium oxalate nephrolithiasis found that individuals on a high calcium diet had less recurrent stones than those on a low calcium diet.[25] The increased dietary calcium presumably binds excessive oxalate within the gut. Therefore, in individuals with a hypercalciuria and nephrolithiasis, it is generally recommended that the majority of calcium should come from food sources. It has been suggested that the increased risk of nephrolithiasis with calcium supplementation can be increased with adequate fluid intake.[26]

Vitamin D

Important advances in the study of vitamin D have led to its acceptance as a hormone with systemic effects well beyond its role in bone physiology, for example, vitamin D supplementation has been shown to prevent acute respiratory infections.[27] The biologic effects of vitamin D are mediated both through genomic and nongenomic pathways involving neuromuscular function in skeletal muscle, small intestine, kidneys, and bones, and as an anti-proliferative, prodifferentiation, and immunomodulatory agent in tissues as diverse as the breast, colon, and prostate gland. The active form of vitamin D, $1,25(OH)_2D_3$, affects calcium and phosphate metabolism in the bone, intestine, and kidney (**Figure 8.4**).[28] The following discussion is limited to the musculoskeletal system.

- **Recommendations for Dietary Intake of Vitamin D and Food Sources**

The recommendations for vitamin D intake are shown in **Table 8.1**.[1] Vitamin D is not widely available in foods, however, egg yolks, cold water fish such as salmon, and cod liver oil contain vitamin D and many foods such as milk are fortified with vitamin D. **Table 8.2** shows vitamin D content of common foods.[28]

- **Label Reading for Vitamin D Intake**

Figure 8.3 shows a food label. The % daily value reflected relates back to 400 International units (IU), therefore if the % daily value as a decimal is multiplied by 400, it will yield the number of IUs in one serving.

- **Source and Function of Vitamin D**

The primary source of vitamin D is from solar UV-B irradiation of skin that triggers the conversion of provitamin D_3 (7-dehydroxycholesterol) to previtamin D_3 and then vitamin D_3 (**Figure 8.4**).[29-32] The latter, plus vitamin D_3 from the diet, is hydroxylated in the liver to form $25(OH)D_3$ (circulating storage form) and in the kidney to $1,25(OH)_2D_3$ (biologically active form). The $1,25(OH)_2D_3$ ligand binds to the vitamin D receptor (VDR) and initiates the biologic function of the target organ: intestine—calcium and phosphorus absorption; muscle—muscle strength and mass; circulating $1,25(OH)_2D_3$ reduces PTH function, both directly and indirectly, by increasing serum calcium. Bone metabolism is also regulated in part by $1,25(OH)_2D_3$ binding to the osteoblast VDR, with the resulting release of biochemical signals and subsequent maturation of osteoclasts.

The latter dissolves bone mineral and matrix, releasing collagen peptides, and calcium into the systemic circulation. With aging, there is a decrease in intestinal calcium absorption which may by mediated by lower circulating levels of $1,25(OH)_2D3$ because of decreased kidney synthesis, intestinal resistance, and increased catabolism of $1,25(OH)_2D3$.[33]

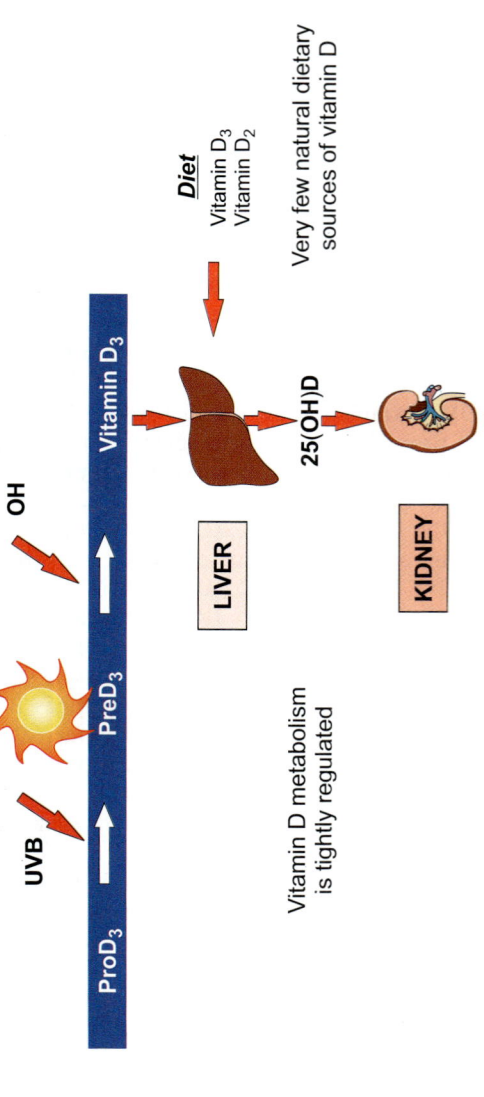

FIGURE 8.4 — Vitamin D, Calcium Absorption, and Bone Health

ProD₃ — UVB → PreD₃ — OH → Vitamin D₃

LIVER

Vitamin D metabolism is tightly regulated

KIDNEY

25(OH)D

Diet
Vitamin D₃
Vitamin D₂

Very few natural dietary sources of vitamin D

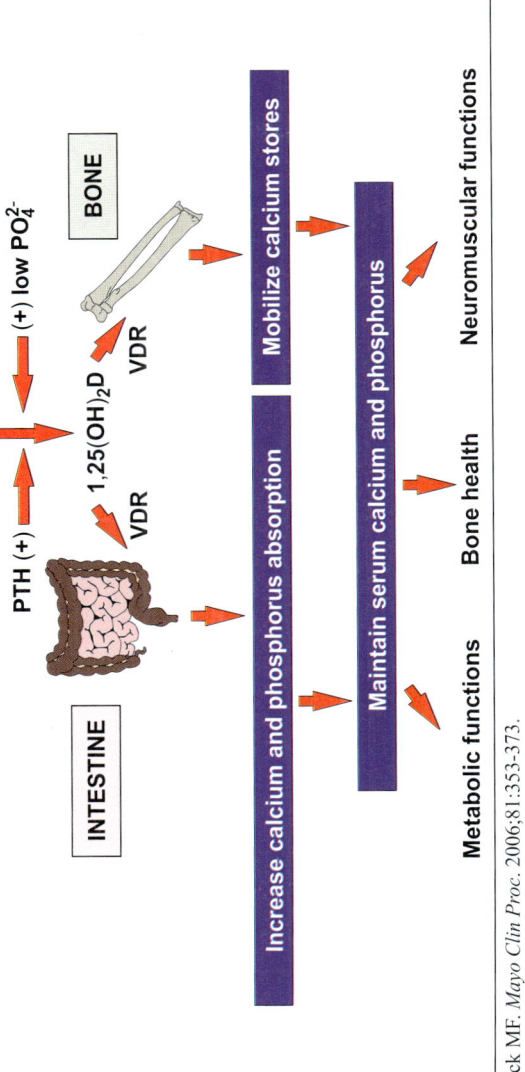

Holick MF. *Mayo Clin Proc.* 2006;81:353-373.

8

165

TABLE 8.2 — Sources of Vitamin D$_2$ and Vitamin D$_3$

Source	Vitamin D Content 1 IU = 25 ng
Natural Sources	
Cod liver oil	~400-1000 IU/teaspoon vitamin D$_3$
Salmon, fresh wild caught	~600-1000 IU/3.5 oz vitamin D$_3$
Salmon, fresh farmed	~100-250 IU/3.5 oz vitamin D$_3$, vitamin D$_2$
Salmon, canned	~300-600 IU/3.5 oz vitamin D$_3$
Sardines, canned	~300 IU/3.5 oz vitamin D$_3$
Mackerel, canned	~250 IU/3.5 oz vitamin D$_3$
Tuna, canned	236 IU/3.5 oz vitamin D$_3$
Shiitake mushrooms, fresh	~100 IU/3.5 oz vitamin D$_2$
Shiitake mushrooms, sun dried	~1600 IU/3.5 oz vitamin D$_2$
Egg yolk	~20 IU/yolk vitamin D$_3$ or D$_2$
Sunlight/UV-B radiation	~20,000 IU equivalent to exposure to 1 minimal erythemal dose in a bathing suit. Thus, exposure of arms and legs to 0.5 minimal erythemal dose is equivalent to ingesting ~3000 IU vitamin D$_3$

Fortified Foods

Fortified milk	100 IU/8 oz usually vitamin D_3
Fortified orange juice	100 IU/8 oz vitamin D_3
Infant formulas	100 IU/8 oz vitamin D_3
Fortified yogurts	100 IU/8 oz usually vitamin D_3
Fortified butter	56 IU/3.5 oz usually vitamin D_3
Fortified margarine	429/3.5 oz usually vitamin D_3
Fortified cheeses	100 IU/3 oz usually vitamin D_3
Fortified breakfast cereals	~100 IU/serving usually vitamin D_3

Pharmaceutical Sources in the United States

Vitamin D_2 (ergocalciferol)	50,000 IU/capsule
Drisdol (vitamin D_2) liquid 8000 IU/mL	

Supplemental Sources

Multivitamin	400, 500, 1000 IU vitamin D_3 or vitamin D_2
Vitamin D_3	400, 800, 1000, 2000, 5000, 10,000, and 50,000 IU

Holick MF. *J Investig Med.* 2011;59(6):872-880.

■ Vitamin D Assessment

Serum $25(OH)D_3$ is the major circulating form of vitamin D and represents the contribution from both dietary intake and skin synthesis and should be the vitamin D form assayed in an individual with normal renal function.[29,34] 25-OH vitamin D levels have been shown to be reduced after elective total hip arthroplasty and it is recommended that the assessment of vitamin D status be completed approximately 6 weeks after the surgery.[35]

■ Optimal Intakes and 25-OH Vitamin D Levels

There is controversy about the optimal amount of daily vitamin D intake and the optimum $25(OH)D_3$ level for bone health.[2,36-38] Like calcium, individuals do not generally get enough vitamin D from the diet and most individuals do not make enough vitamin D in their skin, therefore, the need for supplementation is common. A reasonable guideline is to recommend a total intake of at least approximately 1000-2000 IU per day and aim for a $25(OH)D_3$ level of 100 nmol/L (40 ng/mL).[36] Of note, the Institute of Medicine recommends slightly lower amounts and a target level of 20 ng/ml at a general population level (**Table 8**.1).[1] Over-the-counter vitamin D supplements tend to be variable in their cholecalciferol content, which may confuse vitamin D dosing.[39] If possible, use a supplement marked as meeting US Pharmacopeia (USP) standards should be selected.[39]

■ Vitamin D and Fractures

Vitamin D alone is not effective in preventing fractures (**Figure 8**.3).[5] Meta-analyses of calcium and vitamin D trials have suggested that intakes of at least 700-800 IU of vitamin D per day are necessary for fracture reduction (**Figure 8**.5).[40-43] A subset analysis of the Women's Health Trial found that long-term use of calcium and vitamin D conferred a reduction in the risk of hip fractures.[44] An autopsy study of 675 individuals where secondary causes were excluded demonstrated that a pathological accumulation of osteoid (a marker of vitamin D deficiency) did not occur with a 25(OH) D$_3$ level >75 nmol/L.[45]

■ Vitamin D and Falls

The combination of calcium and vitamin D together lowers the fracture risk in adults >65 years of age.[7] The fracture risk is reduced even in the absence of a significant increase in bone mass. This is attributable to vitamin D associated improvement in muscle strength and balance.[46,47] The mechanisms underlying the effect of vitamin D in the muscle are currently under study (**Figure 8.6**).

■ Vitamin D Toxicity

There are mixed data about the effects of high dose vitamin D related to falls, cancer, and mortality.[48,49] There may be a "u-shaped" relationship between vitamin D and a variety of health outcomes and overzealous supplementation may not be advantageous. There are several prospective trials of vitamin D supplementation related to the effects on blood pressure, cancer, cardiovascular disease, diabetes, falls, and longevity underway.[50] A study where fall incidence and serum 25-OH vitamin D levels were collected as a secondary outcome, found that falls increased as serum 25-OH vitamin D level exceeded 40-45 ng/mL.[51]

8

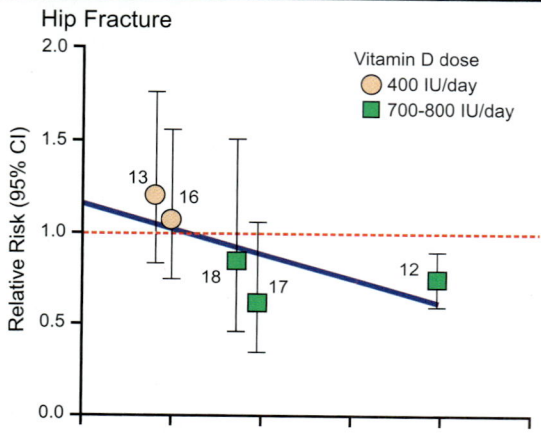

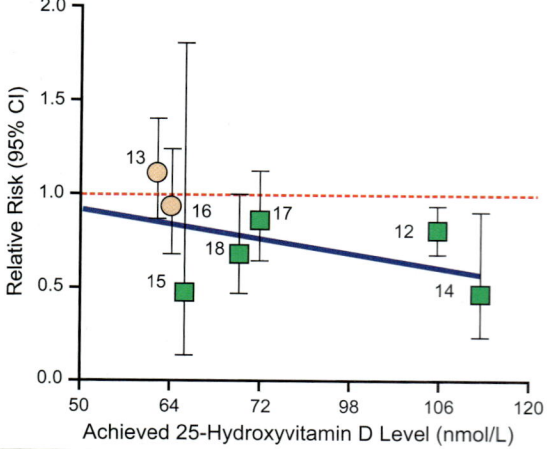

Bischoff-Ferrari HA, et al. *JAMA*. 2005;293(18):2257-2264.

REFERENCES

1. Academies IoMotN. DRIs for Calcium and Vitamin D. National Academy of Sciences; 2010.

2. Ross AC, Manson JE, Abrams SA, et al. The 2011 report on dietary reference intakes for calcium and vitamin D from the Institute of Medicine: what clinicians need to know. *J Clin Endocrinol Metab*. 2011;96(1):53-58.

3. Clinic UOPaT. Tone Your Bones Calcium Calculator. 2003.

4. Mangano KM, Walsh SJ, Insogna KL, et al. Calcium intake in the United States from dietary and supplemental sources across adult age groups: new estimates from the National Health and Nutrition Examination Survey 2003-2006. *J Am Diet Assoc*. 2011;111(5):687-695.

5. Heaney RP, Rafferty K. The settling problem in calcium-fortified soybean drinks. *J Am Diet Assoc*. 2006;106(11):1753, author reply 5.

6. Heaney RP. Absorbability and utility of calcium in mineral waters. *Am J Clin Nutr*. 2006;84(2):371-374.

7. Group D. Patient level pooled analysis of 68 500 patients from seven major vitamin D fracture trials in US and Europe. *BMJ*. 2010;340:b5463.

8. Moyer VA; U.S. Preventive Services Task Force. Vitamin D and calcium supplementation to prevent fractures in adults: U.S. Preventive Services Task Force recommendation statement. *Ann Intern Med*. 2013;158(9):691-696.

9. Thorning TK, Raben A, Thostrup T, et al. Mil, and dairy products: good or bad for human health? An assessment of the totality of scientific evidence. *Food Nutr Res*. 2016;60:32527.

10. Bolland MJ, Avenell A, Baron JA, et al. Effect of calcium supplements on risk of myocardial infarction and cardiovascular events: meta-analysis. *BMJ*. 2010;341:c3691.

11. Bolland MJ, Barber PA, Doughty RN, et al. Vascular events in healthy older women receiving calcium supplementation: randomised controlled trial. *BMJ*. 2008;336(7638):262-266.

12. Bolland MJ, Grey A, Avenell A, et al. Calcium supplements with or without vitamin D and risk of cardiovascular events: reanalysis of the Women's Health Initiative limited access dataset and meta-analysis. *BMJ*. 2011;342:d2040.

13. Li K, Kaaks R, Linseisen J, Rohrmann S. Associations of dietary calcium intake and calcium supplementation with myocardial infarction and stroke risk and overall cardiovascular

8

FIGURE 8.6 — Direct and Indirect Effects of Vitamin D on Muscle

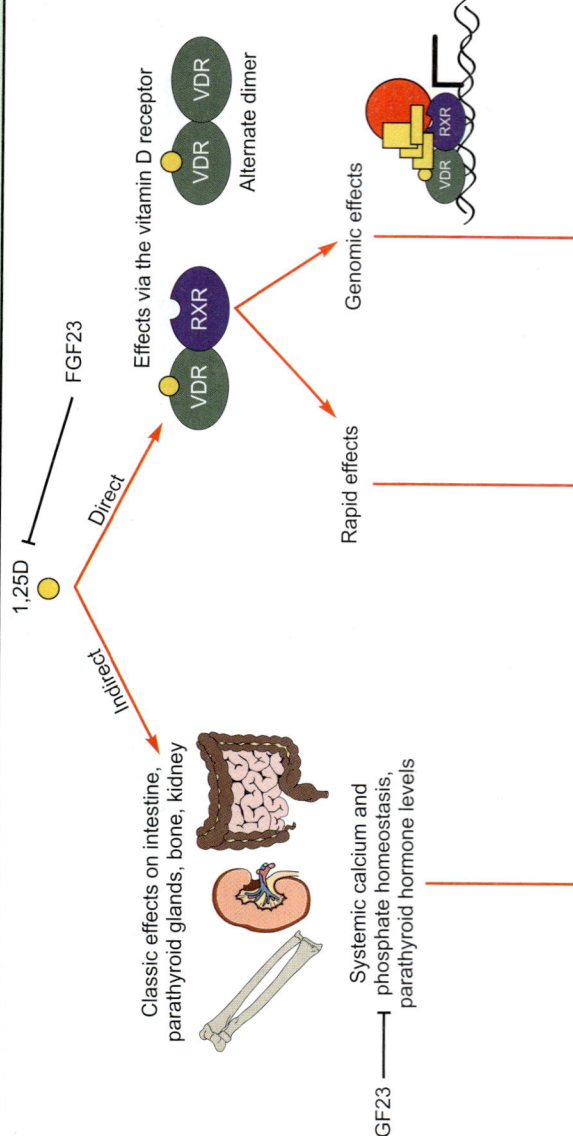

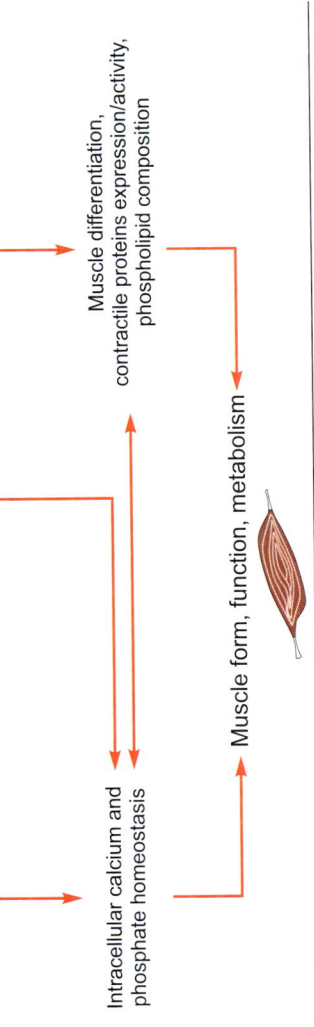

Muscle differentiation, contractile proteins expression/activity, phospholipid composition

Muscle form, function, metabolism

Intracellular calcium and phosphate homeostasis

Data on direct effects come predominantly from in vitro studies and are yet to be confirmed in vivo, where the presence of the VDR is currently under debate.

Girgis CM, et al. *Endocr Rev.* 2013;34(1):33-83.

8

mortality in the Heidelberg cohort of the Europena Prospective Investigation into Cancer and Nutrition Study (EPIC-Heidelberg). *Heart*. 2012;98(12):920-925.

14. Prentice RL1, Pettinger MB, Jackson RD, et al. Health risks and benefits from calcium and vitamin D supplementation: Women's Health Initiative clinical trial and cohort study. *Osteoporos Int*. 2013;24(2):567-580.

15. Paik JM1, Curhan GC, Sun Q, et al. Calcium supplement intake and risk of cardiovascular disease in women. *Osteoporos Int*. 2014;25(8):2047-2056.

16. Samuelson EJ, Booth SL, Fox CS, et al. Calcium intake is not associated with increased coronary artery calcification: the Framingham Study. *Am J Clin Nutr*. 2012 Dec;96(6):1274-1280.

17. Lewis JR, Zhu K, Thompson PL, Prince RL. The effects of 3 years of calcium supplementation on common carotid artery intimal thickness and carotid atherosclerosis n older women: an ancillary study of the CAIFOS randomized controlled trial. *J Bone Miner Res*. 2014;29(3):534-541.

18. Navhavi M, Libby P, Falk E, et al. From vulnerable plaque to vulnerable patient: A call for new definitions and risk assessment strategies: Part I. *Circulation*. 2003;108(14):1664-1672.

19. Lewis JR, Radavelli-Bagatini S, Rejnmark L, et al. The effects of calcium supplementation on verified coronary heart disease hospitalization and death in postmenopausal women: a collaborative meta-analysis of randomized controlled trials. *J Bone Miner Res*. 2015;30(1):165-175.

20. Chung M, Tang AM, Fu Z, Wang DD, Newberry SJ. Calcium intake and cardiovascular disease risk: An updated systematic review and meta-analysis. *Ann Intern Med*. 2016;165(12):856-866.

21. Kopecky SL, Bauer DC, Gulati M, et al. Lack of evidence linking calcium with or without vitamin D supplementation to cardiovascular disease in generally healthy adults: A clinical guidelines from the National Osteoporosis Foundation and the American Society for Preventive Cardiology. *Ann Intern Med*. 2016;165(12):867-868.

22. Jackson RD, LaCroix AZ, Gass M, et al. Calcium plus vitamin D supplementation and the risk of fractures. *N Engl J Med*. 2006;354(7):669-683.

23. Asplin JR, Bauer KA, Kinder J, et al. Bone mineral density and urine calcium excretion among subjects with and without nephrolithiasis. *Kidney Int*. 2003;63(2):662-669.

24. Melton LJ 3rd, Crowson CS, Khosla S, et al. Fracture risk among patients with urolithiasis: a population-based cohort study. *Kidney Int*. 1998;53(2):459-464.

25. Borghi L, Schianchi T, Meschi T, et al. Comparison of two diets for the prevention of recurrent stones in idiopathic hypercalciuria. *N Engl J Med*. 2002;346(2):77-84.

26. Harris SS ,Dawson-Hughes B. Effects of hydration and calcium supplementation on urine calcium concentration in healthy postmenopausal women. *J Am Coll Nutr*. 2015:34 (4):340-346.

27. Martineau AR, Jolliffe DA, Hooper RL, et al. Vitamin D supplementation to prevent acute respirator tract infections: systematic review and meta-analysis of individual participant data. *BMJ*. 201715;356:i6583.

28. Yoshida T, Stern PH. How vitamin D works on bone. *Endocrinol Metab Clin North Am*. 2012;41(3):557-569.

29. Binkley N, Ramamurthy R, Krueger D. Low vitamin D status: definition, prevalence, consequences, and correction. *Rheum Dis Clin North Am*. 2012;38(1):45-59.

30. Heaney RP. The Vitamin D requirement in health and disease. *J Steroid Biochem Mol Biol*. 2005;97(1-2):13-19.

31. Holick MF. High prevalence of vitamin D inadequacy and implications for health. *Mayo Clin Proc*. 2006;81(3):353-373.

32. Holick MF. Vitamin D: a d-lightful solution for health. *J Investig Med*. 2011;59(6):872-880.

33. Veldurthy V, Wei R, Oz L, et al. Vitamin D, calcium homeostasis and aging. *Bone Res*. 2016;18(4):16041.

34. Holick MF, Binkley NC, Bischoff-Ferrari HA, et al. Evaluation, treatment, and prevention of vitamin D deficiency: an Endocrine Society clinical practice guideline. *J Clin Endocrinol Metab*. 2011;96(7):1911-1930.

35. Binkley N, Coursin D, Krueger D, et al. Surgery alters parameters of vitamin D status and other laboratory results. *Osteoporos Int*. 2017;28:1013-1020.

36. Binkley N, Lewiecki EM. Vitamin D and common sense. *J Clin Densitom*. 2011;14(2):95-99.

37. Brouwer-Brolsma EM, Bischoff-Ferrari HA, Bouillon R, et al. Vitamin D: do we get enough? A discussion between vitamin D experts in order to make a step towards the harmonisation of dietary reference intakes for vitamin D across Europe. *Osteoporos Int*. 2013;24(5):1567-1577.

8

38. Heaney RP, Holick MF. Why the IOM recommendations for vitamin D are deficient. *J Bone Miner Res*. 2011;26(3):455-457.

39. Leblanc ES, Perrin N, Johnson JD, Ballatore A, Hillier T. Over-the-counter and compounded vitamin D: is potency what we expect? *JAMA Intern Med*. 2013;173(7):585-586.

40. Bischoff-Ferrari HA, Willett WC, Orav EJ, et al. A pooled analysis of vitamin D dose requirements for fracture prevention. *N Engl J Med*. 2012;367(1):40-49.

41. Bischoff-Ferrari HA, Willett WC, Wong JB, et al. Fracture prevention with vitamin D supplementation: a meta-analysis of randomized controlled trials. *JAMA*. 2005;293(18):2257-2264.

42. Bischoff-Ferrari HA, Willett WC, Wong JB, et al. Prevention of nonvertebral fractures with oral vitamin D and dose dependency: a meta-analysis of randomized controlled trials. *Arch Intern Med*. 2009;169(6):551-561.

43. Tang BM, Eslick GD, Nowson C, et al. Use of calcium or calcium in combination with vitamin D supplementation to prevent fractures and bone loss in people aged 50 years and older: a meta-analysis. *Lancet*. 2007;370(9588):657-666.

44. Prentice RL, Pettinger MB, Jackson RD, et al. Health risks and benefits from calcium and vitamin D supplementation: Women's Health Initiative clinical trial and cohort study. *Osteoporos Int*. 2013;24(2):567-580.

45. Priemel M, von Domarus C, Klatte TO, et al. Bone mineralization defects and vitamin D deficiency: histomorphometric analysis of iliac crest bone biopsies and circulating 25-hydroxyvitamin D in 675 patients. *J Bone Miner Res*. 2010; 25(2):305-312.

46. Girgis CM, Clifton-Bligh RJ, Hamrick MW, et al. The roles of vitamin d in skeletal muscle: form, function, and metabolism. *Endocr Rev*. 2013;34(1):33-83.

47. Michael YL, Whitlock EP, Lin JS, et al. Primary care-relevant interventions to prevent falling in older adults: a systematic evidence review for the U.S. Preventive Services Task Force. *Ann Intern Med*. 2010;153(12):815-825.

48. Melamed ML, Michos ED, Post W, et al. 25-hydroxyvitamin D levels and the risk of mortality in the general population. *Arch Intern Med*. 2008;168(15):1629-1637.

49. Sanders KM, Stuart AL, Williamson EJ, et al. Annual high-dose oral vitamin D and falls and fractures in older women: a randomized controlled trial. *JAMA*. 2010;303(18):1815-1822.

50. Kupferschmidt K. Uncertain verdict as vitamin D goes on trial. *Science*. 2012;337(6101):1476-1478.

51. Smith LM, Gallagher JC, Suiter C. Medium doses of daily vitamin D decrease falls and higher doses of daily vitamin D3 increase falls: a randomized clinical trial [published online ahead of print March 18, 2017]. *J Steroid Biochem Mol Biol*. doi: 10.1016/j.jsbmb.2017.03.015.

8

9 Prevention and Treatment: Pharmacologic Agents

Drug Classes

Based on their effects on bone remodeling, drugs used to prevent and/or treat osteoporosis fall into three main classes:

- Antiresorptive agents:
  - These drugs inhibit osteoclast activity
  - Most of the drugs in clinical practice today are in this category and include:
    - Bisphosphonates
    - Selective estrogen receptor modulators (SERMS) and Tibolone
    - RANKL inhibitor, denosumab
    - Calcitonin
    - Postmenopausal hormone replacement therapy (HT)
- Bone formation stimulants (anabolic agents)
  - These drugs stimulate osteoblast-mediated bone formation.
  - Teriparatide (rhPTH[1-34]) and abaloparatide (PTHrP[1-34]) are approved drugs in this category.
- Strontium ranelate

The mechanism of action of strontium ranelate is not completely understood. It has relatively weak effects on bone remodeling and probably increases bone strength by alteration of bone's material properties.

The antiresorptive and anabolic agents (other than HT preparations) approved for the treatment and/or prevention of postmenopausal osteoporosis are listed in **Table 9.1**.

TABLE 9.1 — Agents Approved for the Treatment or Prevention of Postmenopausal Osteoporosis[a]

Drugs	Dose/Method of Administration	Reduction in Risk of Fracture	Side Effects	Approved Indications
Bisphosphonates				
Alendronate	35-70 mg weekly or 5-10 mg daily (oral)	Vertebral and hip fracture	Esophagitis, myalgias	Treatment and prevention
Alendronate/ cholecalciferol	70 mg/2800 IU or 70 mg/ 5600 IU once weekly (oral)	Vertebral and hip fracture	Esophagitis, myalgias	Treatment
Ibandronate	150 mg monthly (oral)	Vertebral fracture	Esophagitis, myalgias	Treatment and prevention
	3 mg every 3 months (IV)	Vertebral fracture	Arthralgias/myalgias, low-grade fever	Treatment
Risedronate	5 mg/day, 35 mg/week, or 75 mg on 2 consecutive days each month (oral), 150 mg/month	Vertebral and composite end point of nonverte-bral fracture	Esophagitis, myalgias	Treatment and prevention
Zoledronic acid	5-mg infusion once a year (IV)	Vertebral, nonvertebral, and hip fracture	Arthralgias/myalgias, low-grade fever, atrial fibrillation	Treatment and prevention

Parathyroid Hormone			
Abaloparatide (PTHrP[1-34])	80 mcg SC daily	Vertebral and nonvertebral	Hypercalcemia	Treatment
Teriparatide (rhPTH[1-34])	20 mcg SC daily	Vertebral and nonvertebral	Hypercalcemia	Treatment
RANKL Inhibitor			
Denosumab	60 mg every 6 mo (SC)	Vertebral and hip fracture	Possible skin reactions ± increase in infections	Treatment
Selective Estrogen Receptor Modulator			
Raloxifene	60 mg daily (oral)	Vertebral fracture	Hot flashes, nausea, DVT, leg cramps	Treatment and prevention
Salmon Calcitonin Preparations			
Calcitonin-salmon	200 IU/mL (100 IU every other day) (IM/SC)	Vertebral fracture	Nausea, injection-site reaction, flushing	Treatment
Calcitonin-salmon	200 IU/inh daily (intranasally)	Vertebral fracture	Nasal adverse effects	Treatment
Strontium Ranelate			
Strontium ranelate	2 g once daily (oral)	Vertebral and hip fracture	Nausea, diarrhea	Treatment

[a] All agents approved for treatment have demonstrated efficacy in reducing fractures as determined in randomized, placebo-controlled trials with fracture as the primary end point.

9

General Guidelines for Pharmacologic Interventions

Internationally, the pharmacologic therapies most often used for osteoporosis include the bisphosphonates alendronate, ibandronate, risedronate, and zoledronic acid; parathyroid hormone analogues teriparatide and abaloparatide; strontium ranelate (not FDA approved in the United States); denosumab; and raloxifene. All of these agents have been shown to reduce the risk of vertebral fracture. Some of these have been shown to also reduce the risk of nonvertebral fractures, in some cases, including hip fracture. Large randomized, placebo-controlled studies suggest that there is a 30% to 86% reduction in the risk of vertebral fractures and a 16% to 43% reduction in the risk of nonvertebral fractures with pharmacologic treatment.[1,2]

A number of general recommendations can be made regarding pharmacologic therapy for osteoporosis:

- Bisphosphonates are usually considered first-line treatment for osteoporosis, particularly because of their positive effects on vertebral, nonvertebral, and hip fractures, and lower cost.
- Second-line options include denosumab, raloxifene, strontium ranelate (in countries where available), and teriparatide.
- Because of its higher cost and the inconvenience of a daily injection, teriparatide use is often confined to high-risk patients, those with fractures and in those with glucocorticoid-induced osteoporosis.
- Largely in the light of the WHI study results and the availability of many other efficacious compounds, HT is no longer be considered first-line therapy and is not approved in the United States as a treatment for osteoporosis.
- Combination use of antiresorptive drugs is generally not recommended because there is

no current evidence of additional antifracture benefits, and there may be an increased risk of side effects and the oversuppression of bone turnover.

Patients who are deemed appropriate candidates for pharmacologic therapy include men and women who have experienced a fragility fracture, those with osteoporotic range bone mass by hip or spine DXA, persons with low bone mass (osteopenia) meeting a FRAX threshold ($\geq$3% for hip and $\geq$20% for major osteoporotic fracture, based on NOF recommendations; outside of the United States, different thresholds have been proposed), and selected individuals without low bone mass but more high fracture risk due to risk states such as glucocorticoids (see also *Chapter 11*).

Bisphosphonates

■ **Pharmacology**
Bisphosphonates are synthetic compounds that have a nonhydrolyzable P-C-P bond that adheres strongly to hydroxyapatite crystals of bone. There are two side chains:
- One binds to bone mineral
- One determines potency (nitrogen molecule).

9

The first generation of bisphosphonates, which are seldom used anymore, include:
- Clodronate
- Etidronate
- Pamidronate (nitrogen-containing molecule or aminobisphosphonates)

The second generation of aminobisphosphonates include:
- Alendronate
- Risedronate

Third-generation aminobisphosphonates include:
- Ibandronate
- Zoledronic acid

Potency of the drugs depends on the length and structure of the side chain (**Figure 9.1**).

It appears the bisphosphonates protect bone via the following pathways:
- Decrease in the differentiation and recruitment of osteoclast precursor cells. This decreases the number of mature active osteoclasts.

FIGURE 9.1 — Bisphosphonates: Chemistry

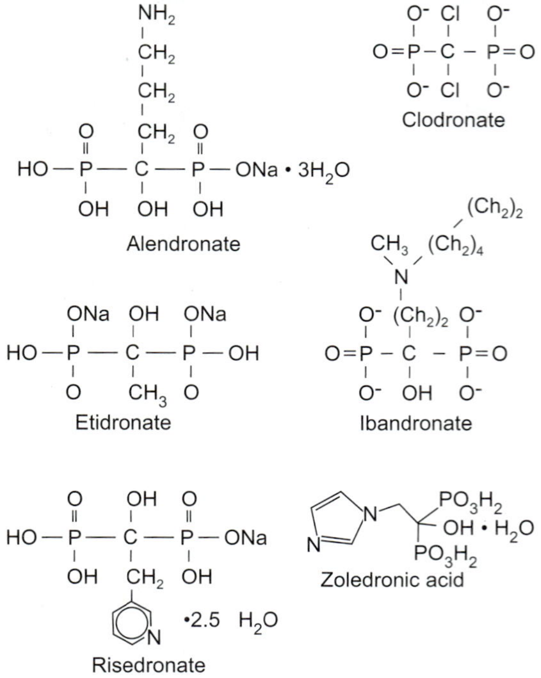

Diez-Perez A. *Maturitas*. 2002;43(suppl 1):S19-S26 and Zometa [package insert]. East Hanover, NJ; Novartis Pharmaceuticals Corporation; 2012.

- Inhibition of integrins. The integrins are the main component of the seal that attaches the osteoclast to the bone surface. The seal facilitates the acid milieu below the osteoclast, which results in "old bone" being resorbed.[3]
- Activation of the caspase system that results in the inhibition of the mevalonate pathway (involved in cholesterol production and statin activity) and the blocking of proteins responsible for the cytoskeletal organization of the osteoclast and for osteoclast cell proliferation and apoptosis (**Figure 9.2**). [4]
- As noted previously, osteoblasts are responsible for the early activation and recruitment of osteoclast precursors, via the RANK-RANKL system. This is inhibited by the aminobisphosphonates.
- Aminobisphosphonates inhibit the apoptosis of osteocytes.

Absorption of oral bisphosphonates is around 1% to 3% of the dose and is decreased by food or calcium (see section below on delayed-release risedronate, which may be taken with food). Calcium binds the drug in the gut. Bisphosphonates are released slowly from the skeleton and residence of the bisphosphonates in the skeleton is very prolonged. About 30% to 50% of the absorbed dose adheres to the active bone surfaces and the rest is excreted in urine.

■ Efficacy of Available Bisphosphonates

Alendronate

Alendronate effectively inhibits osteoclast-mediated bone resorption at doses that do not impair bone mineralization. Alendronate is approved for both the prevention and treatment of osteoporosis in postmenopausal women and for the treatment of osteoporosis in men.

FIGURE 9.2 — Bisphosphonate Cellular and Molecular Mechanisms of Action

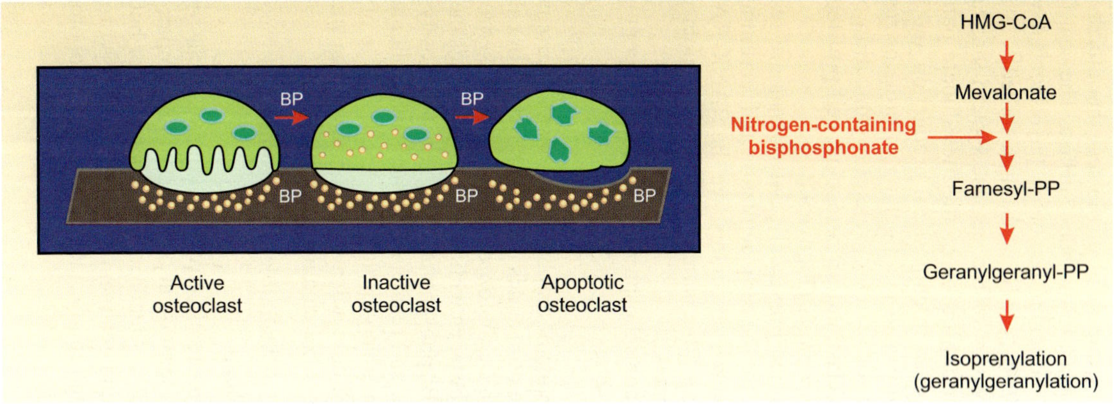

Daily Dosing

A significant reduction in hip, wrist, and vertebral fractures was demonstrated in the 36- to 48-month Fracture Interventional Trial (FIT), a randomized, double-blind, placebo-controlled study of alendronate in women with low femoral neck BMD without vertebral fracture and in a cohort of women with existing vertebral fracture.[5] Dosage was 5-mg alendronate daily for 2 years and 10 mg daily for the following year.

The results showed the following reductions in the relative risk (RR) of fracture:

- 53% for the hip
- 48% for radiographic vertebral fracture
- 45% for clinical vertebral fractures.

Another placebo-controlled study of postmenopausal women with low BMD showed a 47% reduction in the risk of nonvertebral fractures after 1 year of 10-mg alendronate daily.[6]

A post hoc analysis of data from older women in FIT study shows that alendronate is effective in reducing the risk of symptomatic osteoporotic fractures across the spectrum of ages.[7]

Once-Weekly Dosing

Once-weekly alendronate 35 mg appears therapeutically equivalent to alendronate 5 mg once daily and once-weekly alendronate 70 mg equivalent to alendronate 10 mg daily.[8-10] Given the easier adherence to once weekly vs daily therapy for most patients, there is now very little residual use of daily alendronate.

There have been two 12-month trials comparing once-weekly alendronate 70 mg with once-weekly risedronate 35 mg in postmenopausal women with low BMD.[11-13] There were significantly greater increases in BMD at all sites measured in the alendronate group compared with those randomized to risedronate (**Figure 9.3**). There were also greater reductions in markers of bone turnover with alendronate compared with risedronate and the tolerability was similar. The

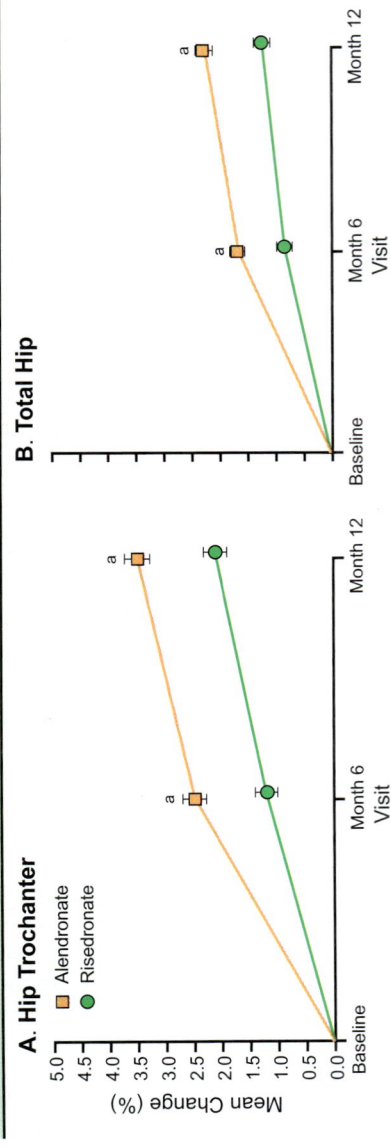

FIGURE 9.3 — Comparison of Change From Baseline to 12 Months in Hip Trochanter, Total Hip, Femoral Neck, and Lumbar Spine BMD in Once-Weekly Treatment With Alendronate or Risedronate

A. Hip Trochanter

B. Total Hip

188

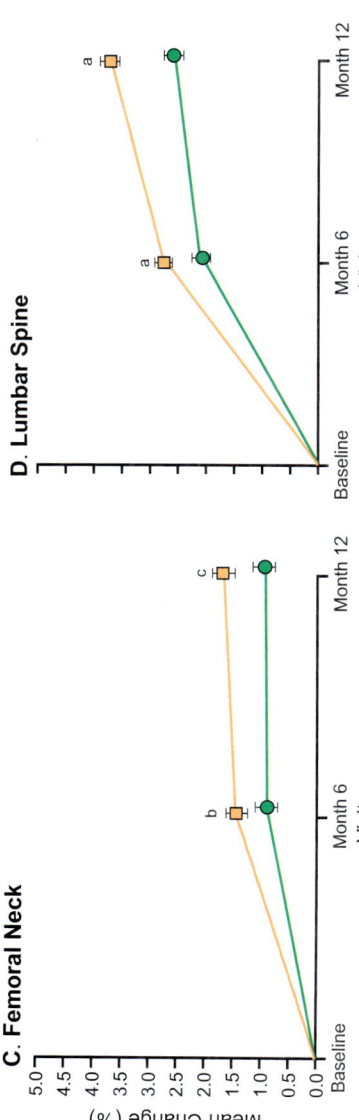

C. Femoral Neck

D. Lumbar Spine

In the Fosamax Actonel Comparison Trial (FACT) in 1053 postmenopausal women with low BMD, once-weekly alendronate 70 mg resulted in significantly greater increases in hip trochanter BMD (*A*), total hip BMD (*B*), femoral neck BMD (*C*), and lumbar spine BMD (*D*) than once weekly risedronate 35 mg. In the subsequent, double-blind extension of the FACT in which patients continued with their original randomized treatment for an additional 1 year, alendronate produced greater increases from baseline in BMD than did risedronate at all other BMD sites after a total of 2 years' treatment. After 2 years, there were no differences in occurrence or discontinuations due to upper GI adverse events.

a *P* <0.001. b *P* <0.05. c *P* <0.01.

Rosen CJ, et al. *J Bone Miner Res.* 2005;20:141-151.

9

studies were not powered to demonstrate differences in fracture reduction and, to date, no studies with sufficient statistical power have demonstrated fracture rate differences between bisphosphonates.

Discontinuation of Treatment

A double-blind extension to the original large alendronate trial compared the effects of discontinuing alendronate treatment after 5 years vs continuing for 10 years in postmenopausal women who had been treated with alendronate in the FIT study (called the FLEX study).[14] Patients were randomized to continue their alendronate regimen (5 mg/day or 10 mg/day) for an additional 5 years or switched to placebo. The cumulative 10-year risk of nonvertebral fractures was not significantly different between those continuing and discontinuing alendronate after 5 years (**Figure 9.4**). However, there was a significantly lower risk of clini-

---

FIGURE 9.4 — Fracture Risk Reduction Comparing 5 Years (Alendronate/Placebo) vs 10 Years of Alendronate (5 mg/10 mg) in the Fracture Intervention Trials Long-Term Extension (FLEX) Study

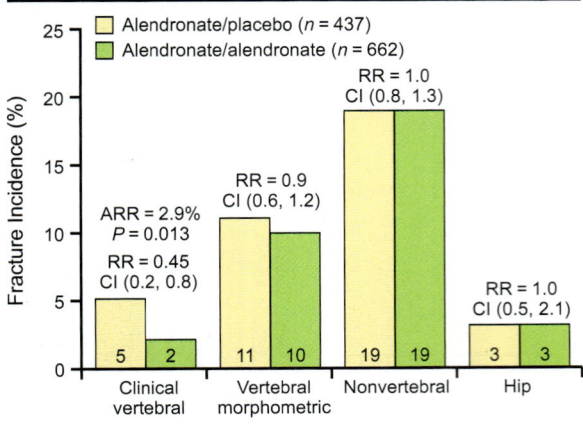

Black DM, et al. *JAMA*. 2006;296(24):2927-2938.

cally recognized vertebral fractures in the group that continued alendronate, but no significant risk reduction difference for morphometric vertebral fractures among those continuing alendronate compared with those who stopped. A subsequent analysis suggested that women with femoral neck T-score of ≤ -2.5 at the time of entry into the extension study continued to receive fracture benefit from alendronate.[15] This finding plus the limited sample size to detect differences in fracture risk temper the suggestion that 5 years may be somewhat equivalent to 10 years of alendronate in terms of fracture risk reduction at certain sites.

Glucocorticoid-Induced Osteoporosis

Alendronate significantly increases BMD at the hip, spine, and trochanter compared with placebo and reduced the risk for vertebral fractures in an extension to the original study.[16,17] Bisphosphonates have vertebral antifracture efficacy similar to their use in postmenopausal osteoporosis in the prevention and treatment of glucocorticoid-induced osteoporosis (**Figure 9.5**).[18] Therapy for glucocorticoid-induced osteoporosis generally should be maintained as long as the patient remains on supra-physiologic glucocorticoid doses (also see *Chapter 11*).

Approved Dosage and Administration

The recommended doses of alendronate for the *prevention* of osteoporosis in postmenopausal women are 5 mg/day or 35 mg once weekly, while the recommended doses for the *treatment* of osteoporosis are 10 mg/day or 70 mg once weekly.

- Each dose should be taken with 6 to 8 oz of plain water (mineral water or well water should not be used with bisphosphonate administration), on arising, at least one half hour before breakfast. The patient should remain sitting up or erect for at least 30 minutes to 1 hour.
- Alendronate is also available as buffered effervescent solution. It is taken once weekly with a smaller amount of water than required with

FIGURE 9.5 — Meta-analysis Comparing Fracture Risk Reduction Due to Alendronate and Risedronate in PMO and GIOP

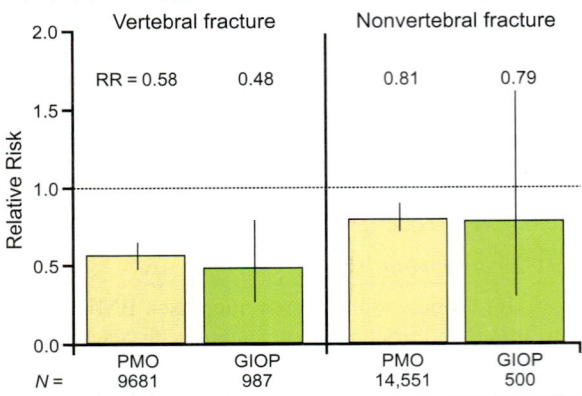

Key: GIOP, glucocorticoid-induced osteoporosis; PMO, postmenopausal osteoporosis.

Kanis JA, et al. *Health Technol Assess*. 2007;11(7):1-231.

tablets. It contains the same-strength ingredient (alendronate sodium 70 mg) as once-weekly alendronate and it appears to be bioequivalent to alendronate 10 mg/daily.

- Calcium supplements and antacids interfere with absorption of alendronate; thus they should be taken at least 30 minutes later.
- No dosage adjustment is necessary for the elderly or for patients with mild-to-moderate renal insufficiency. Alendronate should be avoided in patients with an estimated GFR <30 mg/min.

Alendronate is also available as a preparation in combination with vitamin D, in a single tablet containing 70-mg alendronate and either 2800-IU or 5600-IU cholecalciferol (vitamin D_3) for once-weekly administration and is approved for treatment of osteoporosis in postmenopausal women.

Risedronate

Risedronate is a second-generation amino-bisphosphonate approved for the *prevention* and *treatment* of postmenopausal osteoporosis. Risedronate suppresses biochemical markers of bone modeling. Bone formed during risedronate treatment is histologically normal. Animal studies have demonstrated that risedronate preserves vertebral trabecular architecture.[19] Several long-term clinical studies that included repeated bone biopsies have shown that risedronate provided sustained and homogeneous benefits on bone mineralization and maintained architecture for up to 5 years.[20]

Daily Dosing

Risedronate has been studied in a number of randomized controlled clinical trials. Based on these trials:

- Risedronate 5 mg daily has been shown to significantly increase the BMD of the spine and hip in women with established osteoporosis within and beyond 5 years of menopause.[21] Increases in BMD are measurable within 6 months of starting treatment.
- Risedronate significantly reduced the cumulative incidence of new vertebral fractures in patients by 41% over 3 years and by 65% after the first year in women with prevalent fractures.[22] The comparable reduction in vertebral fractures in a large multinational study was 49% after 3 years of treatment and 61% within the first year following the initiation of the trial. Nonvertebral fractures were reduced by 30% to 40%.[23]
- A 5-mg daily dose of risedronate compared with placebo for 3 years significantly reduced the vertebral fracture risk in established osteoporosis.[22,24] The relative reduction of new vertebral fractures in women with at least one vertebral fracture at baseline was 41% and 39% for nonvertebral fractures. In women with at least

two baseline vertebral fractures, the risk of new vertebral fractures was reduced by 49%. In a blinded continuation of one of these studies on a subset population, the antifracture efficacy of risedronate was maintained for 5 years.[24-26]

- In the Hip Intervention Program (HIP) trial, the incidence of hip fracture among those assigned risedronate was 2.8% vs 3.9% among the placebo group, a significant 30% RRR.[27] In the 70- to 79-year-old group, the incidence of hip fracture among risedronate recipients was 1.9% vs 3.2% among those taking placebo, a significant 40% RRR. The incidence of hip fractures among those at least 80 years old, selected primarily for nonskeletal risk factors, and not requiring a BMD inclusion criteria, did not differ significantly at 4.2% among those assigned to risedronate vs 5.1% among those assigned to placebo. The authors concluded that risedronate significantly reduced the risk of hip fracture among elderly women with confirmed osteoporosis but not among elderly women selected for risk factors other than low BMD.

Once-Weekly and Twice-Monthly Dosing

Risedronate 35 mg once weekly or 75 mg on 2 consecutive days each month was therapeutically equivalent to risedronate 5 mg daily in the treatment of postmenopausal women with osteoporosis.[28,29] Similar to alendronate, almost all risedronate is administered on a weekly or monthly basis (150 mg orally), predicated by patient convenience and adherence considerations.

Glucocorticoid -Induced Osteoporosis

Risedronate prevents vertebral and nonvertebral bone loss in patients initiating or continuing long-term glucocorticoid therapy.[30,31] This was associated with a 70% reduction in vertebral fracture risk in a post hoc pooled analysis.[32]

- Recommended dosages of risedronate for *prevention or treatment* of osteoporosis in postmenopausal women are 5 mg daily, 35 mg once weekly, 75 mg on 2 consecutive days each month, or 150 mg orally every month.

- As with other bisphosphonates, the intestinal absorption of risedronate is very low. The absorption of risedronate is decreased by 55% if the medication is taken <30 minutes before breakfast or 2 hours after dinner. Consequently, risedronate is recommended to be taken at least 30 minutes before the first food or drink of the day (except water), without lying down for 30 minutes afterward. No dosage adjustment is necessary for the elderly or for patients with mild-to-moderate renal insufficiency. A delayed-release form of risedronate 35 mg per week is approved and can be taken with food.

- Risedronate 35 mg is also available co-packaged with 1250-mg calcium carbonate (500 mg elemental calcium), which is supplied in a blister pack containing four 35-mg risedronate tablets and 24 calcium carbonate tablets to provide a full 28-day course of therapy. The 35-mg risedronate tablet is taken once weekly followed by 6 days of calcium carbonate.

9

Ibandronate

Ibandronate, a third-generation oral bisphosphonate, has twice the in vitro potency of risedronate and ten times the potency of alendronate. Because of its high affinity to bone and the prolonged effect on bone after being absorbed onto the bone surface, various daily and intermittent regimens of ibandronate for both the treatment and prevention of osteoporosis have been evaluated and are approved.[33, 34]

Ibandronate is approved by the FDA as 2.5 mg oral once-daily or 150 mg once-monthly dosing regimens for the *treatment and prevention* of postmenopausal osteoporosis and, more recently, 3 mg IV every 3 months administered over 15 to 30 seconds for treatment only. Ibandronate has not been shown to reduce hip fracture.[35-38]

Oral Treatment

- The 3-year Oral Ibandronate Osteoporosis Vertebral Fracture Trial in North America and Europe (BONE) study assessed the anti-fracture effects of oral ibandronate 2.5 mg daily or 20 mg every other day for 12 doses every 3 months in postmenopausal women with low BMD at the lumbar spine and one to four vertebral fractures.[39] After 3 years, both the daily and intermittent oral ibandronate regimens produced significant reductions of 62% and 50%, respectively, in the RR of new vertebral fractures compared with placebo. Both ibandronate regimens also produced significant RRR of new or worsening clinical vertebral fractures (49% and 48% for daily and intermittent, respectively) compared with placebo. There was no significant difference in anti-fracture efficacy between the daily and intermittent ibandronate regimens. All ibandronate-treated patients experienced significantly greater increases in BMD (6.5% and 5.7% vs 1.3% for placebo) at the lumbar spine and total hip (3.4% and 2.9% vs -0.7% for placebo) from baseline. These BMD increases were progressive over the 3-year treatment period with a significant difference observed at 6 months and at all later time points compared with placebo.
- A 2-year Monthly Oral Ibandronate In Ladies (MOBILE) study (**Figure 9.6**).[40,41] In addition, 150 mg once monthly was found to be superior) to 2.5 mg daily in terms of the increase in lumbar spine BMD, the primary end point. The 150-mg regimen consistently produced greater increases in BMD than the 100 mg monthly and daily regimens.

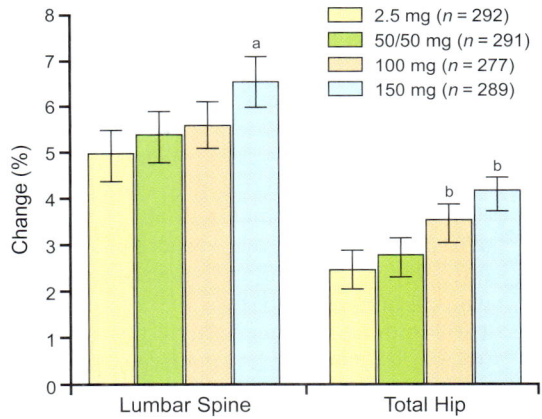

The 2-year MOBILE study compared the safety and efficacy of three ibandronate monthly regimens vs daily ibandronate in the treatment of postmenopausal osteoporosis. A total of 1609 women who were ≥5 years menopausal with lumbar spine T-score between -2.5 and -5 received one of the following ibandronate regimens: 50/50 mg monthly (50 mg doses on 2 consecutive days), 100 mg once monthly, 150 mg once monthly, or 2.5 mg once daily.

[a] *P*<0.001 vs daily treatment.
[b] *P*<0.05 vs daily treatment.

Adapted from Reginster JY, et al. *Ann Rheum Dis.* 2006;65:654-661.

Three different regimens of oral daily (0.5 mg, 1 mg, 2.5 mg) ibandronate were also shown to prevent bone loss in a placebo-controlled study of postmenopausal women without osteoporosis at baseline.[42] After 2 years, oral ibandronate produced a dose-related and sustained maintenance or increase in BMD at the lumbar spine and hip (total hip, femoral neck, trochanter), as well as dose-related reduction in the rate of bone turnover. The greatest BMD increases were observed with the 2.5 mg dose, which produced significant BMD gains in lumbar spine and total hip BMD (3.1% and 1.8%, respectively) compared with placebo at 24 months.

Intravenous Treatment

Several randomized, placebo-controlled trials have evaluated IV ibandronate once every 3 months:

- One placebo-controlled trial assessed the efficacy of ibandronate 0.5 mg, 1 mg, or 2 mg every 3 months in the prevention of osteoporosis in postmenopausal women without osteoporosis at baseline.[43] After 1 year, ibandronate produced dose-dependent and statistically significant gains in lumbar spine BMD of 2.5%, 1.8%, and 1.0% in the groups receiving 2 mg, 1 mg, and 0.5 mg ibandronate, respectively, compared with a loss of 0.4% in the women in the placebo group. In addition, all three doses of ibandronate produced significantly better gains in BMD at the hip than placebo. The greatest gains in spine and hip BMD occurred in the women with osteopenia receiving the 2-mg dose.

- Another study assessed 1 mg or 2 mg every 3 months in postmenopausal, osteoporotic women. After 1 year, the 2-mg dose provided significantly greater efficacy than the 1-mg dose.[44] Lumbar spine BMD increased by 5.0% and 2.8% in the 2-mg and 1-mg groups, respectively, and decreased by 0.04% in the placebo group.

Oral vs Intravenous

The therapeutic equivalence of IV ibandronate 2 mg every 2 months or 3 mg every 3 months with 2.5 mg daily was assessed in postmenopausal women with osteoporosis.[35] After 1 year, lumbar spine BMD increases were 5.1% among patients receiving 2 mg of ibandronate every 2 months, 4.8% among patients receiving 3 mg every 3 months, and 3.8% in women who received daily oral ibandronate. Hip BMD increases (all sites) were also greater in the groups receiving IV ibandronate than in the group receiving oral ibandronate.

Dosage and Administration

The recommended doses of ibandronate for the treatment and prevention of osteoporosis in postmenopausal women are:

- 150 mg PO once monthly taken at least 60 minutes before the first food or drink (other than water) of the day or before taking any oral medication or supplements, including calcium, antacids, or vitamins with a full glass of plain water; the patient must remain in an upright position for at least 60 minutes
- 3 mg injected IV once every 3 months (for treatment only)
- Patients should receive supplemental calcium or vitamin D if dietary intake and/or vitamin D stores are inadequate.

Zoledronic Acid

Zoledronic acid is the most potent bisphosphonate studied to date. IV zoledronic acid was initially approved for the treatment of multiple myeloma and for patients with bone metastases from solid tumors and is approved by the FDA and EMA for *treatment and prevention* of postmenopausal osteoporosis and osteoporosis in men.

Approval was based on the results of the 3-year, placebo-controlled Health Outcomes and Reduced Incidence with Zoledronic Acid Once Yearly (HORIZON) Pivotal Fracture Trial.[45,46] At 3 years, zoledronic acid treatment reduced the risk of morphometric vertebral fractures by 70% compared with placebo (**Figure 9.7**). Zoledronic acid also reduced the risk of hip fracture by 41% compared with placebo. There also were significant reductions in the incidence

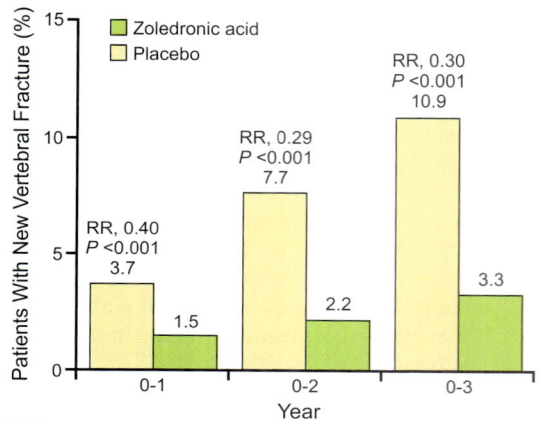

FIGURE 9.7 — Incidence of Morphometric Vertebral Fracture With Once-Yearly IV Zoledronic Acid or Placebo

Adapted from Black DM, et al. *N Engl J Med.* 2007;356:1809-1822.

of nonvertebral fractures (25%), all clinical fractures (33%), and clinical vertebral fractures (77%) in the zoledronic acid group compared with the placebo group. In addition, there were significant improvements in BMD and bone turnover markers in the zoledronic acid-treated patients.

The HORIZON Recurrent Fracture Trial uniquely assessed the efficacy of zoledronic acid for the prevention of new clinical fractures in patients who had recently suffered a hip fracture, a previously under-studied group.[47,48] In addition, the safety analysis included all-cause mortality. The first infusions were administered within 90 days after surgical repair of a hip fracture. The rate of any new clinical fracture in the zoledronic acid group was 8.6% compared with 13.9% in the placebo group, a significant absolute risk reduction of 5.3% and a relative reduction of 35% (**Table 9.2**). The RR reductions in new clinical vertebral (46%)

TABLE 9.2 — Reduction in the Risk of Fractures and All-Cause Mortality With Zoledronic Acid

Variable	Placebo ($n = 1062$)	Zoledronic Acid ($n = 1065$)	Hazard Ratio	P Value
Fracture –N (cumulative %)				
Any	139 (13.9)	92 (8.6)	0.65	0.001
Nonvertebral	107 (10.7)	79 (7.6)	0.73	0.03
Hip	33(3.5)	23 (2.0)	0.70	0.18
Vertebral	39 (3.8)	21 (1.7)	0.54	0.02
Death –N (cumulative %)	141 (13.3)	101 (9.6)	0.72	0.01

Adapted from Lyles KW, et al. *N Engl J Med*. 2007;357(18):1799-1809.

9

and new clinical nonvertebral fractures (27%) in the zoledronic acid group were also significantly lower than in the placebo group (**Table 9.2**). In terms of all-cause mortality, 9.6% of patients in the zoledronic acid group and 13.3% of patients in the placebo group (13.3%) died, a significant RR reduction of 28%.

In an extension of the HORIZON trial, women randomized to zoledronic acid experienced, on average, 18 fewer days of back pain compared with placebo over the course of the trial.[49] The back pain among women randomized to zoledronic acid vs placebo resulted in 11 fewer days of limited activity. Women randomized to zoledronic acid were about 6% less likely to experience 7 or more days of back pain or limited activity owing to back pain. Women randomized to zoledronic acid were significantly less likely to experience 7 or more bed-rest days owing to a fracture and 7 or more limited-activity days owing to a fracture. Reductions in back pain with zoledronic acid were independent of incident fracture.

Data from extension studies suggest slight but statistically significantly greater BMD gains and greater fracture risk reductions comparing three once-yearly doses of zoledronic acid with six once-yearly doses.[50] Similarly, the point estimates of fracture risk reduction for patients in the recurrent fracture trial who received three infusions were slightly better than those who received only one infusion.[51] Given its potency and protracted skeletal retention, the similarity of the data between shorter vs longer courses of zoledronic acid has encouraged some clinicians to consider dosing less frequent than once every year in patients at lower fracture risk.

Dosage and Administration

Zoledronic acid is indicated for *treatment* or prevention of osteoporosis in postmenopausal women.
- Zoledronic acid should be administered through a separate vented infusion line as a single 5-mg infusion once a year given over no less than

15 minutes. For prevention, it is given every 2 years.
- Do not allow the solution come in contact with any calcium or divalent cation-containing solutions.
- Administration of zoledronic acid is not recommended in patients with severe renal impairment (creatinine clearance <35 mL/min).
- Serum creatinine should be monitored before each dose.
- All patients should have a routine oral exam by the prescriber prior to treatment.
- Patients must be appropriately hydrated prior to the administration of zoledronic acid.
- Patients must be adequately supplemented with calcium and vitamin D.
- Zoledronic acid, as well as all bisphosphonates, passes through the placental barrier and is taken up by the fetal skeleton. Women of childbearing potential should be advised of the potential hazard to the fetus and avoid becoming pregnant.
- Patients receiving zoledronic acid for malignancy considerations (different brand name) should not receive it for osteoporosis (both of which are zoledronic acid).

Other Bisphosphonates

A number of other bisphosphonates have been developed and are used for the treatment of malignant diseases of bone and Paget's disease of bone. These include:
- Clodronate
- Tiludronate
- Pamidronate
- Etidronate

Etidronate is prescribed outside of the United States (not FDA approved) for the treatment of osteoporosis. Etidronate should be prescribed cyclically as follows:

- 400 mg daily for 2 weeks taken on an empty stomach or midafternoon (ie, between lunch and dinner)
- No calcium supplements for the 2 weeks of treatment
- Dosage is repeated every 3 months.

Bisphosphonates Side Effects and Potential Safety Issues

Long-term trials with bisphosphonates revealed no long-term safety issues, and there were few links between potential side effects and duration of treatment. A number of definite and potential bisphosphonate side effects have been identified

Gastrointestinal

Although side effects in clinical trials were generally minimal (abdominal pain, nausea, dyspepsia, constipation, and diarrhea), about 3% of patients in a postmarketing surveillance study developed esophageal ulcers on alendronate. Of the 211 esophageal reactions to alendronate reported worldwide, 36 were serious; in about half the reported cases, the drug had not been taken in accordance with the prescribing information (with inadequate amount of water or patient did not remain upright for 30 minutes or more). In one study, a 3-fold increase in risk for GI problems was due mostly to comorbid conditions and other factors.[52] Alendronate 70 mg once weekly was not associated with any increase in endoscopic lesions in the upper GI tract relative to placebo.[53] Like alendronate, risedronate may cause upper GI side effects. In the studies of oral regimens of ibandronate, the incidence of upper GI events was low with no differences observed across all treatment arms.[42] Dyspepsia, nausea, and abdominal pain were the most commonly reported upper GI events with oral ibandronate.

Two methodologically different analyses of the same large database reached opposite conclusions about whether alendronate and other oral bisphosphonates may be associated with esophageal cancer.[54,55]

Osteonecrosis of the Jaw (ONJ)

In addition to osteoporosis, bisphosphonates, particularly the potent IV nitrogen-containing agents, have long been used to treat metabolic bone diseases and skeletal events associated with metastatic neoplasms. There have been reports of ONJ in patients receiving IV regimens of bisphosphonates for malignancy with rate estimates of 1% to 10% (**Figure 9.8**).[56] A small number of patients with osteoporosis using oral or IV bisphosphonates have also been reported to develop ONJ.[57,58] In most cases, poor dental hygiene, dental procedures, or poor-fitting dentures were associated risk factors. The risk of ONJ among patients with osteoporosis treated with bisphosphonates is very low, estimated at between 1 in 10,000 and 1 in 100,000 person years of bisphosphonate exposure. Preventive measures, such as oral examination and treatment of

9

FIGURE 9.8 — Osteonecrosis of the Palatal Torus in a Patient With Osteoporosis Taking Alendronate

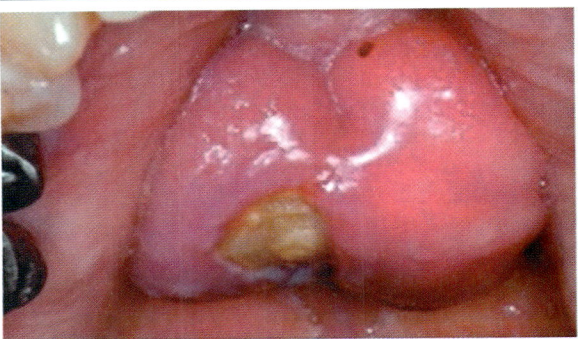

Woo SB, et al. *Ann Intern Med*. 2006;144(10):753-761.

dental infection prior to initiating bisphosphonate therapy, should be encouraged together with maintenance of good oral hygiene. US dental societies have issued position papers encouraging bisphosphonate users to still seek dental care, dentists to provide that care, and suggesting strategies to mitigate these concerns.[59]

Atypical Femoral Fractures

There have been a number of case reports and case series, and a growing number of observational studies reporting associations between atypical fractures at the subtrochanteric region of the femur in bisphosphonate-treated patients.[60-62] Common features of these atypical fractures include prodromal pain, occurrence with minimal/no trauma, a thickened diaphyseal cortex, and transverse fracture pattern (**Figure 9**.**9**). The American Society of Bone and Mineral Research has developed a case definition for this outcome.[63] A large registery-based study and retrospective analyses of phase 3 trials of bisphosphonates, however, did not show an increased risk of subtrochanteric fractures with bisphosphonate use. The number of atypical subtrochanteric fractures in association with bisphosphonates is an estimated one per 1000 per year.[64]

Physicians should remain vigilant in assessing their patients on long-term bisphosphonates and advise them of this potential risk. Although bisphosphonate use rarely may be associated with atypical subtrochanteric fractures, the risk-benefit ratio still remains favorable for use of bisphosphonates to prevent fractures over the short to moderate term.[65] Some physicians have considered the long-term skeletal safety, coupled with the known skeletal retention of bisphosphonates, and the data on fracture risk reduction near equivalence comparing shorter- vs longer-term bisphosphonate courses as a justification for a "drug holiday" after a protracted period of therapy, such as a 5-year course of oral alendronate.

Post Infusion Acute Phase Reactions

Zoledronic acid is associated with transient postinfusion symptoms of arthralgias, myalgia, and pyrexia, sometimes presenting as flu-like illness. This so-called acute phase reaction can affect up to 15% of patients and appears more frequent during the first infusion. The most common adverse events with IV Ibandronate are mild to moderate joint pain, back pain, flu-like symptoms, abdominal pain, and inflammation of the nose and throat. These tend to occur during the week after the injection.

Renal Impairment

There were transient >0.5 mg/dL increases in the serum creatinine level in 1.3% of women in the zoledronic acid group at 9 to 11 days postinfusion. By 30 days postinfusion, the levels returned to normal in the majority of women.[50] Although clinical trials of oral bisphosphonates have not detected significant renal impairment, bisphosphonates should be avoided in patients with estimated GFRs less than 30-35 mL/min. Secondary analyses of the risedronate studies showed that even among patients with moderate renal insufficiency, bisphosphonates continue to be efficacious.[66]

Atrial Fibrillation

There was an increase in serious atrial fibrillation events in one zoledronic acid study (1.3% on zoledronic acid vs 0.5% in placebo, respectively).[45] However, no difference was observed in the occurrence of stroke or death due to stroke. These findings were surprising since in the 559 patients who underwent ECGs there was no difference in the prevalence of atrial fibrillation in the zoledronic acid and placebo groups.[50] Further, this finding was not evident in a review of existing trials and the FDA concluded that this was not a class effect of bisphosphonates.[67]

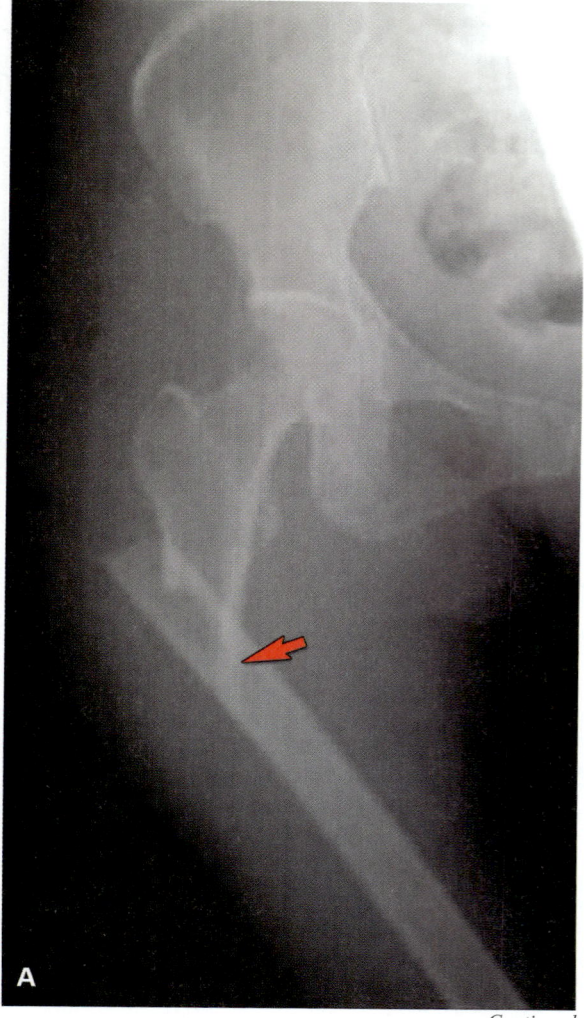

A

Continued

FIGURE 9.9 — *Continued*

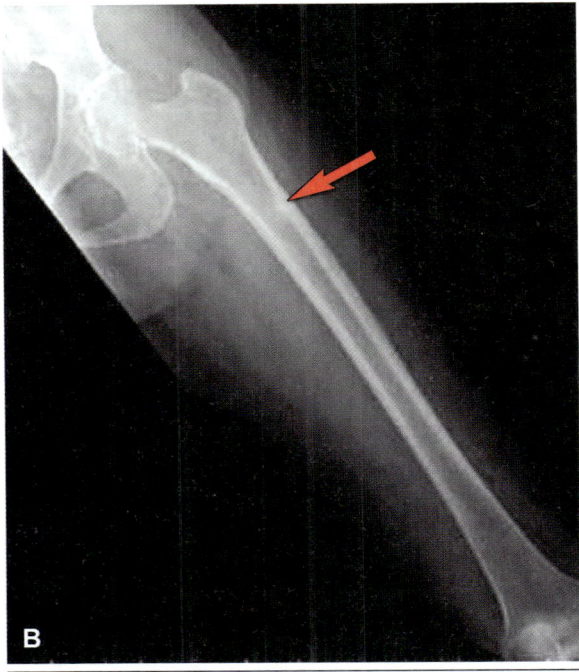

Atypical femoral subtrochanteric fracture demonstrating medial beaking *(short arrow) (A)*; prodromal stress fracture in the contralateral leg of the same patient *(long arrow) (B)*.

Goh SK, et al. *J Bone Joint Surg Br*. 2007;89(3):349-353.

Fracture Healing

It appears that bisphosphonates in the doses usually prescribed for osteoporosis prevention/treatment are safe to use in subjects who have recently experienced fracture. However, because of the lack of efficacy of zoledronic acid within 2 weeks postfracture compared with later zoledronic acid treatment in patients with hip fracture, zoledronic acid should not be administered until at least 2 weeks after the fracture.[68]

Arthralgias and myalagias may occur insidiously in patients on oral as well as IV bisphosphonates. These are typically reversible on discontinuation of therapy.

Anterior uveitis has rarely been reported associated with bisphosphonates.[69]

Hypocalcaemia is seen, particularly with the potent IV preparations. Patients should have sufficient serum calcium and vitamin D stores before IV administration. Pre-treatment with ergocalciferol 100,000 IUs was given prior to IV zoledronic acid in the Recurrent Fractures Trial.[48]

Bisphosphonates in Children

Off-label bisphosphonate treatment is sometimes used in some children with osteogenesis imperfecta, idiopathic juvenile osteoporosis, and glucocorticoid-induced osteoporosis.[70] Given the long-term skeletal retention of these drugs along with insufficient evidence about the effects of exposure of a fetus to a bisphosphonate, these agents should be used with considerable caution in premenopausal women of child-bearing potential (also see *Chapter 11*).

Selective Estrogen Receptor Modulators (SERMs)

■ Raloxifene

Systemic Beneficial Effects

Raloxifene is a SERM that binds to ER (primarily ERα) in bone, breast, and uterine cells and acts as an estrogen antagonist in breast and uterus but an agonist in bone and the cardiovascular system. There is a 60% to 70% reduction in breast cancer risk with use of raloxifene and the FDA has approved its use for reduction in risk of invasive breast cancer in postmenopausal women with osteoporosis, postmenopausal women at high risk for invasive breast cancer, and for *treatment* and *prevention* of osteoporosis in postmenopausal women.

Beneficial effects of raloxifene on serum lipids are about half those of conjugated estrogens 0.625 mg but without uterine-stimulating effects.[71] Animal studies suggest that the lipid-lowering effect of raloxifene compared with conjugated estrogen is not associated with a reduction in coronary artery atherosclerosis.

Bone Efficacy

- In early postmenopausal women, raloxifene prevents postmenopausal bone loss at the spine and hip (2.7% at the lumbar spine and 2.4% at the femoral neck after 3 years of 60 mg raloxifene daily) but to a lesser degree than that following estrogen therapy (ET) and HT.
- It reduces biochemical markers of bone turnover to premenopausal levels. This probably results from the blocking of cytokines that promote osteoclast differentiations.
- A 3-year trial (Multiple Outcomes of Raloxifene Evaluation [MORE]) resulted in a 30% reduction of vertebral fractures in women with prevalent fractures and a 50% reduction of spinal fractures in women without prevalent fractures.[72-74] No reduction in nonvertebral or hip fractures was shown. The paradox between the modest increase in lumbar BMD but also a robust decrease in the incidence of vertebral fracture has been attributed to the ability of raloxifene to inhibit perforation of the trabecular plates, thereby maintaining the structural integrity (and strength) of the microarchitecture of cancellous bone. This may be a mechanism of action common to all antiresorptive agents.
- In two 5-year trials, the North American and European Prevention Trials and the Study of Tamoxifen and Raloxifene (STAR), raloxifene was found to maintain BMD, reducing the likelihood of onset of osteoporosis.[75,76] In an extension of the MORE study (Continuing Outcomes Relevant to Evista [CORE]), there was no differ-

9

ence in incidence of new nonvertebral fractures after 8 years except in women with preexisting fractures.[77] CORE demonstrated the long-term safety of raloxifene.

Side Effects

- Hot flash symptoms are provoked in up to a third of previously asymptomatic menopausal women on a 60-mg once-daily dose of raloxifene vs only about 3% of women on continuous combined HT with estrogen and progesterone
- No cognitive impairment in postmenopausal women was observed compared with placebo-treated controls but also no improvement in cognitive status (although in two studies, raloxifene-treated women did better than controls in two tests of verbal memory and attention).[78]
- Although rare, the risk of thromboembolic disease (venous thrombosis and pulmonary embolism) is increased; similar to that seen with HT.[79] In women at increased risk of cardiovascular disease, raloxifene increased the risk of fatal stroke but not all strokes.[80]

Dosage and Administration

Raloxifene is approved for:

- *Treatment* and *prevention* of osteoporosis in postmenopausal women
- Reduction in risk of invasive breast cancer in postmenopausal women with osteoporosis
- Reduction in risk of invasive breast cancer in postmenopausal women at high risk for invasive breast cancer.

The daily dose of raloxifene is 60 mg orally.

■ Tibolone

Tibolone is a synthetic steroid described as a tissue-specific drug that acts through its metabolites on estrogen, progesterone, and androgen receptors.

Although used in Asia, Australia, Central/South America and Europe, tibolone is not currently approved in the United States.

Efficacy

Tibolone prevents bone loss in perimenopausal and late postmenopausal women. One study in *recently menopausal* women found significant increases from baseline in BMD of the spine with daily tibolone doses of 0.625 mg, 1.25 mg, and 2.5 mg (1.1%, 2.0%, and 2.6%, respectively) compared with a loss of 2.3% in patients on placebo.[81] A 2-year, placebo-controlled study in *older* postmenopausal women (mean age 66 years) reported increases from baseline in lumbar spine BMD of 5.9% with tibolone 1.25 mg/day and 5.1% with tibolone 2.5 mg/day.[82] In *osteoporotic* postmenopausal women (mean age 65 years) with previous fractures, tibolone 2.5 mg/day significantly increased the BMD at the spine and the femoral neck by 6.9% and 4.5%, respectively.

A 10-year, prospective, nonrandomized trial found that tibolone 2.5 mg/day treatment resulted in increases from baseline in lumbar spine and femoral neck BMD of 4.8% and 3.7%, respectively, compared with decreases of -8.5% and -8.95%, respectively in the control population.[83] A 2-year, randomized, double-blind, study in postmenopausal women compared tibolone 1.25 mg/day or 2.5 mg/day with continuous combined HT (E_2/NETA) and found that the proportion of responders (women whose BMD was >2% after 2 years) was higher in those who received HT (98.5%) than with tibolone, either 2.5 mg (85.7%) or 1.25 mg (89.0%).[84] Tibolone has been shown to reduce vertebral and nonvertebral fractures.[85]

Tibolone's clinical profile also includes:
- Reducing hot flashes and symptoms of urogenital atrophy
- Inhibiting the endometrium
- Lowering elevated levels of cholesterol, triglycerides, and low-density lipoprotein (LDL) cholesterol.

Side Effects

- A slight increase in venous thromboembolism comparable to that associated with HT has been observed.[86]
- High-density lipoprotein (HDL) may experience a reduction of up to 30%.[87] This has, however, been explained by an increase in the efficiency of the HDL–reverse cholesterol transport system and, in animal studies, has not been associated with an increase in atherogenic disease.
- Available data on the long-term safety of tibolone indicates that there may be an increased risk of breast cancer in women who had already suffered from breast cancer in the past and, in a separate trial, an increase in the risk of stroke in women whose mean age was over 60 years.[88,89] The long-term intervention on fractures with tibolone (LIFT) study was discontinued because of an increased risk of stroke during an average of 2.4 years of the trial with a hazard ratio of 2.59.[85,90] After nearly 3 years of therapy, there were 25 (1.11%) strokes (ischemic plus hemorrhagic) in the tibolone group compared with 11 (0.49%) in the placebo group (significant HR = 2.3), and 44 (2.1%) vertebral fractures (based on a semiquantitative reading of the radiographs) compared with 85 (4.1%) on placebo (significant HR = 0.5).

Dosage and Administration

The daily oral dose of tibolone is 2.5 mg.

RANKL Inhibitors

■ Denosumab

Denosumab is the first biological treatment approved for the management of osteoporosis. It is indicated for the treatment of postmenopausal women with osteoporosis at increased risk for fracture, defined as a history of osteoporotic fracture, or multiple risk factors for fracture. This high-affinity, high-specificity, human monoclonal antibody binds to and inhibits RANKL, an essential differentiation and activation factor for osteoclasts, thereby resulting in a reduction of bone resorption (**Figure 9.10**).

Efficacy

The effects of denosumab and alendronate on BMD and biochemical markers of bone turnover were compared in a 12-month, active-controlled trial in post-menopausal women with low BMD.[91] Women received various dosages of denosumab either every 3 months or every 6 months, open-label oral alendronate 70 mg once weekly, or placebo.

All denosumab regimens resulted in increases in BMD at the lumbar spine (3.0% to 6.7% compared with an increase of 4.6% with alendronate and a loss of 0.8% with placebo). Denosumab also increased total hip BMD (1.9% to 3.6% compared with an increase of 2.1% with alendronate and a loss of 0.6% with placebo), and at the distal third of the radius (0.4% to 1.3% compared with decreases of 0.5% with alendronate and 2.0% with placebo.) The most effective dose of denosumab in the group receiving the every-3-month regimen appeared to be 30 mg; for the patients on the every-6-month regimen, 60 mg appeared optimal. The maximum mean percentage reduction in levels of serum C-telopeptide was 88% among the denosumab groups compared with 6% percent in the placebo group. The duration of the decrease was dose-dependent.

The Fracture Reduction Evaluation of Denosumab in Osteoporosis Every 6 Months (FREEDOM) trial found that compared with placebo, denosumab significantly reduced the incidence of new radiographic vertebral fractures by 68% (**Figure 9.11**).[92] In addition, denosumab significantly reduced the risk of nonvertebral and hip fractures, and new clinical fractures (**Table 9.3**). After 36 months, denosumab treatment was associated with a relative increase in BMD of 9.2% at the lumbar spine and 6.0% at the total hip compared with placebo. Denosumab also decreased serum

216

FIGURE 9.10 — Mechanism of Action of RANKL Inhibitor Denosumab

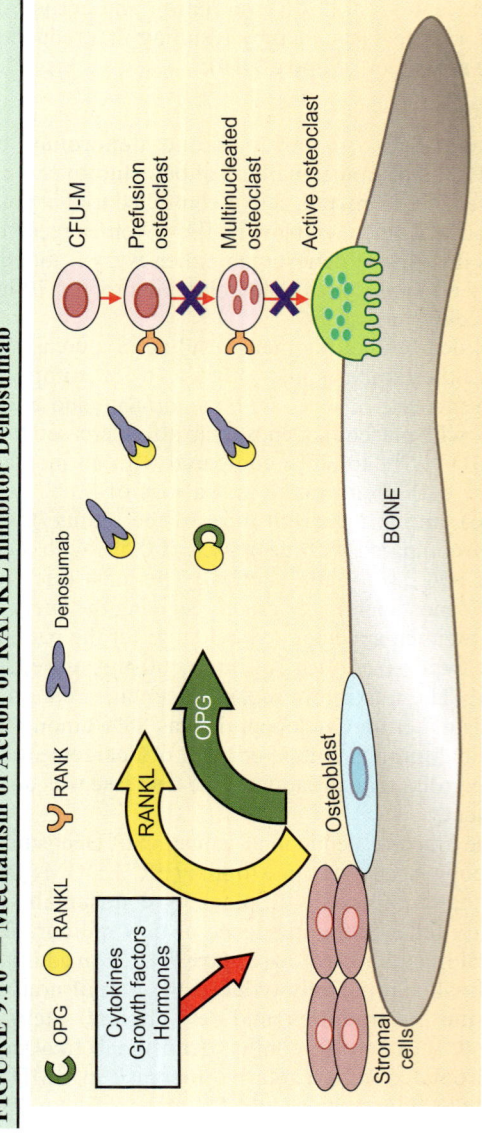

Boyle WJ, et al. *Nature*. 2003;423(6937):337-342.

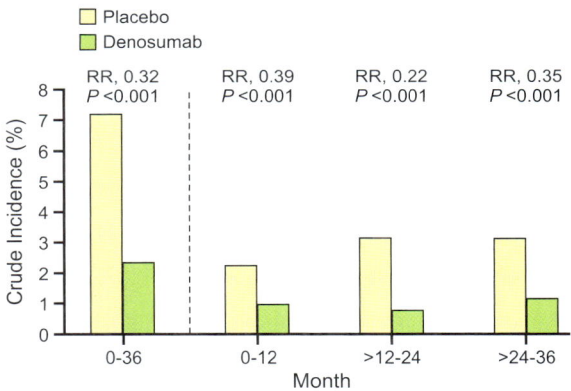

In the FREEDOM trial, denosumab 60 mg every 6 months significantly ($P<0.001$) reduced the incidence of new radiographic vertebral fracture by 68% (7.2% in the placebo group vs 2.3% in the denosumab group).

Risk ratios (RRs) are for patients treated with denosumab compared with patients who received placebo.

Cummings SR, et al. *N Engl J Med*. 2009;361(8):756-765.

C-telopeptide levels by 72% at 36 months compared with placebo.

Results of a phase 2, 4-to-6 year trial of denosumab indicated that there were continuous gains in BMD over 6 years and continued suppression of bone resorption, as demonstrated by bone markers.[93,94] During the first year after withdrawal of treatment, there was a rapid increase of biochemical turnover markers to above baseline levels and a decrease in BMD values to near baseline levels.

A post hoc analysis of the data from the FREEDOM trial evaluated fracture incidence in women with known risk factors for fractures, includ-

TABLE 9.3 — Effect of Denosumab Compared With Placebo on the Risk of Fractures at 36 Months[a]

Outcome	Denosumab n (%)	Placebo n (%)	Relative Risk or Hazard Ratio (95% CI)	P Value
Primary End Point				
New vertebral fractures	86 (2.3)	264 (7.2)	0.32 (0.26-0.41)	<0.001
Secondary End Points				
Nonvertebral fractures	238 (6.5)	293 (8.0)	0.80 (0.67-0.95)	0.01
Hip fractures	26 (0.7)	43 (1.2)	0.60 (0.37-0.97)	0.04
Other Fracture End Points				
New clinical vertebral fractures	29 (0.8)	92 (2.6)	0.31 (0.20-0.47)	<0.001
Multiple (≥2) new vertebral fractures	23 (0.6)	59 (1.6)	0.39 (0.24-0.63)	<0.001

[a] The percentages of new and multiple new vertebral fractures are calculated for 3702 subjects in the denosumab group and 3691 in the placebo group who underwent spinal radiography at baseline and during at least one visit after baseline. The percentages of nonvertebral, hip, and new clinical vertebral fractures are cumulative Kaplan–Meier estimates for 3902 subjects in the denosumab group and 3906 in the placebo group.

Cummings SR, et al. *N Engl J Med*. 2009;361(8):756-765.

ing multiple and/or moderate or severe prevalent vertebral fractures, aged 75 years or older, and/or femoral neck BMD T-score of ≤-2.5.[95] Compared with placebo, denosumab significantly reduced the risk of new vertebral fractures in women with multiple and/or severe prevalent vertebral fractures (16.6% placebo vs 7.5% denosumab). Similarly, denosumab significantly reduced the risk of hip fractures in subjects aged 75 years or older (2.3% placebo vs 0.9% denosumab) or with a baseline femoral neck BMD T-score of ≤2.5 (2.8% placebo vs 1.4% denosumab). These risk reductions in higher-risk individuals were consistent with those seen in those at lower risk of fracture.

Patients who completed the FREEDOM study and who did not discontinue or miss >1 dose of an investigational product were eligible to enter an extension study, which evaluated the long-term safety of denosumab.[96] Data from the first 5 years of the extension are currently available, representing up to 8 years of denosumab exposure for women who received 3 years of denosumab in the parent trial and continued in the extension. Of the 5928 women who were eligible for the extension, 4550 were enrolled. All participants received open-label denosumab subcutaneously every 6 months with daily calcium and vitamin D supplementation. Sustained reductions in serum CTx and P1NP were observed through year 5 of the extension. Compared to FREEDOM baseline, mean percentage changes in lumbar spine, total hip, and femoral neck BMD at each time point were significantly greater than those observed at the previous time point. Following 5 years of treatment in the extension study, totaling up to 8 years of treatment, mean percentage changes in BMD were 18.4% for lumbar spine, 8.3% for total hip, 7.8% for femoral neck, and 3.5% for 1/3 radius (P <0.05 in all instances). The incidence of new vertebral and nonvertebral fractures remained low throughout the extension. In conclusion, data from the ongoing long-term extension study of FREEDOM demonstrated that continued use of denosumab for up to 8 years resulted in sustained reduction in bone turnover, continued gains in BMD at each time point, and continued low yearly fracture incidence rates.

Side Effects

Denosumab was generally well tolerated in clinical trials, with an overall safety profile similar to that with placebo or active comparator. Decreases in serum calcium levels to <8.5 mg/dL have been reported in 0.4% women receiving placebo and in 1.7% women receiving denosumab at the month 1 visit. The nadir in serum calcium level occurs at approximately day 10 after denosumab dosing in subjects with normal renal function. A significantly higher number of women treated with denosumab developed epidermal and dermal adverse events (eg, dermatitis, eczema, and rashes), with these events reported in 8.2% with placebo and 10.8% with denosumab groups. Most of these events were not specific to the injection site. During the FREEDOM trial, there was no increase in the risk of cancer, infection, cardiovascular disease, delayed fracture healing, or hypocalcemia.[92] Osteonecrosis of the jaw in women treated with denosumab has been reported during the osteoporosis clinical trial program and in oncology studies; no cases were reported during FREEDOM trial. At least one case of an atypical fracture has also been associated with denosumab. Compared with placebo or alendronate, a slight increase in a small number of infections, particularly of the skin (cellulitis and erysipelas), has been seen in some but not all denosumab studies.[97-99]

In the long-term extension study of FREEDOM, the overall safety profile of denosumab remained consistent through 8 years of treatment, with incidence rates for all adverse events during the extension period being similar to or lower than rates observed in the active treatment group of the parent trial.

Discontinuing Treatment

The Denosumab And Teriparatide Administration (DATA) study was a 24-month, open-label, randomized controlled trial, where postmenopausal women were randomized 1:1:1 to receive either teriparatide 20-μg subcutaneously daily, denosumab 60-mg subcutaneously every 6 months, or both medications.[100] Enrolled patients were 36+ months since last menses and at high fracture risk. The study demonstrated that concurrent treatment with teriparatide and denosumab increased spine and hip BMD more than either drug alone.

Patients who completed DATA were invited to participate in DATA-Switch, which investigated the safety and efficacy of the transition from teriparatide or combined teriparatide/denosumab to denosumab monotherapy and the transition from denosumab to teriparatide monotherapy.[101] Since teriparatide administration is limited to 2 years, switching from combination therapy to teriparatide was not investigated. In this study, switching from teriparatide to denosumab increased bone mineral density at all sites measured, whereas switching from denosumab to teriparatide resulted in transient bone loss at the hip and spine and progressive bone loss at the radius shaft (**Figure 9.12**). Thus, DATA-Switch demonstrated that although denosumab further increases BMD when used after either teriparatide or combination therapy, teriparatide did not adequately prevent bone loss after denosumab.

Following DATA-Switch, 4 years after their initial enrollment, patients were counseled to follow-up with their physician and strongly consider re-initiation of osteoporosis therapy. Patients who completed all visits were asked to return for BMD assessment at least 12 months following completion of the study.[102] At the follow-up visit, the consequences of discontinuing treatment without further antiresorptive therapy were assessed, as well as the efficacy of physician-prescribed antiresorptive medications. Of the 69 women who completed all DATA and DATA-Switch visits, 50 returned for follow-up assessments. Of these patients, 28 were prescribed an antiresorptive agent between the end of DATA-Switch and their follow-up, and 22 were not. Changes in BMD between the end of DATA-Switch and follow-up assessment in treated vs untreated women are shown in **Figure 9.13**. All patients who

FIGURE 9.12 — DATA-Switch: Mean Percent Change in BMD From Baseline to 48-Months

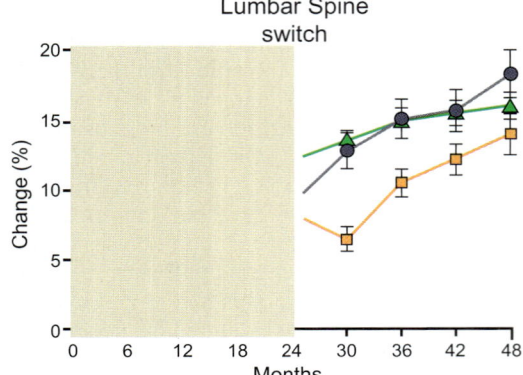

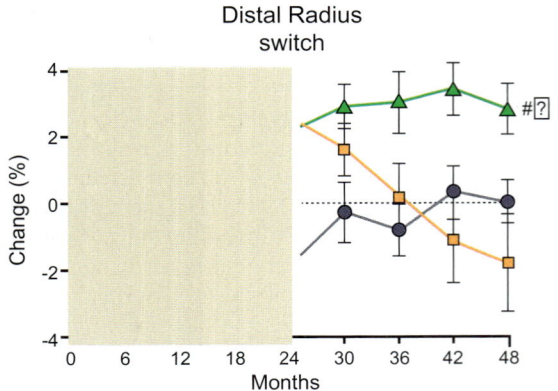

Continued

FIGURE 9.12 — *Continued*

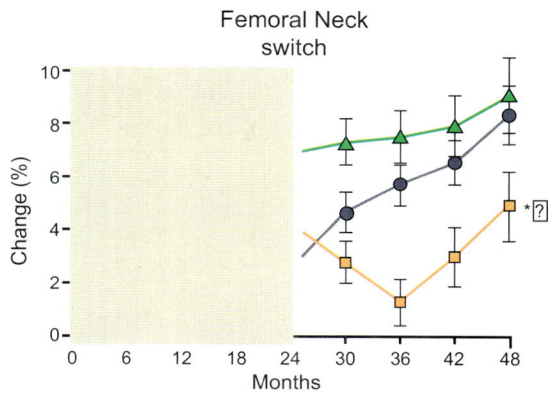

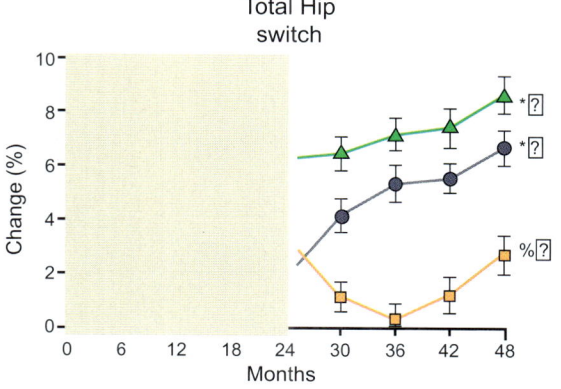

Key: COMBO, combination treatment; DMAB, denosumab; TPTD, teriparatide.

[a] *P*<0.05 vs both other groups.
[b] *P*<0.01 vs both other groups.
[c] *P*<0.0005 vs both other groups.

Adapted from Leder BZ, et al. *Lancet*. 2015;386(9999):1147-1155.

FIGURE 9.13 — DATA-Follow-Up: Percent Change in BMD in Patients Who Did or Did Not Receive Consolidation Therapy

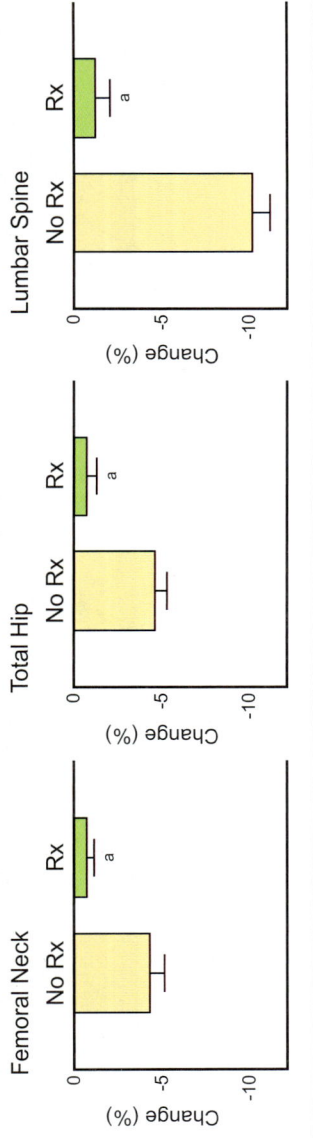

Key: No Rx, did not receive therapy; Rx, received therapy.

[a] *P*<0.001 *vs* No Rx.

Adapted from Leder BZ, et al. *Bone.* 2017;98:54-58.

received no follow-up therapy experienced a reduction in spine BMD, 82% experienced bone loss for femoral neck, and 86% experienced bone loss for total hip. A comparison of the changes in BMD among untreated women who discontinued denosumab vs teriparatide at the end of DATA-Switch are shown in **Figure 9.14**. Spine BMD changes were similar among those discontinuing denosumab and teriparatide; however, femoral neck BMD and total hip BMD decreased significantly more in patients discontinuing denosumab compared to teriparatide. Among women who did receive follow-up treatment, there were no significant differences in the change in BMD between those discontinuing denosumab vs teriparatide at the femoral neck, total hip, or lumbar spine. These results highlight the importance of avoiding a "drug holiday" in postmenopausal osteoporotic women who are being treated with either teriparatide or denosumab.

In summary, the DATA studies established that bone loss is inevitable in postmenopausal women if treatment with teriparatide or denosumab are discontinued and no alternative osteoporosis medication is initiated. However, there are few reasons to stop denosumab therapy, since treatment remains effective over prolonged periods of time, intolerance is uncommon, and there is no clear risk associated with the duration of therapy.[103] Therefore, it is recommended that physicians do not discontinue denosumab therapy in patients once their BMD has stabilized and they are no longer at high-risk of fracture. Patients should be encouraged to continue treatment long-term, and if treatment must be discontinued, then appropriate steps should be taken to protect against rapid bone loss and acute fracture risk, such an initiating an appropriate replacement antiresorptive agent.

Dosage and Administration

- The recommended dose of denosumab is 60 mg administered as a single subcutaneous injection once every 6 months in the upper arm, the upper thigh, or the abdomen.

FIGURE 9.14 — DATA-Follow-Up: Percent Change in BMD in Untreated Patients Who Discontinued Teriparatide vs Denosumab at the End of DATA-Switch

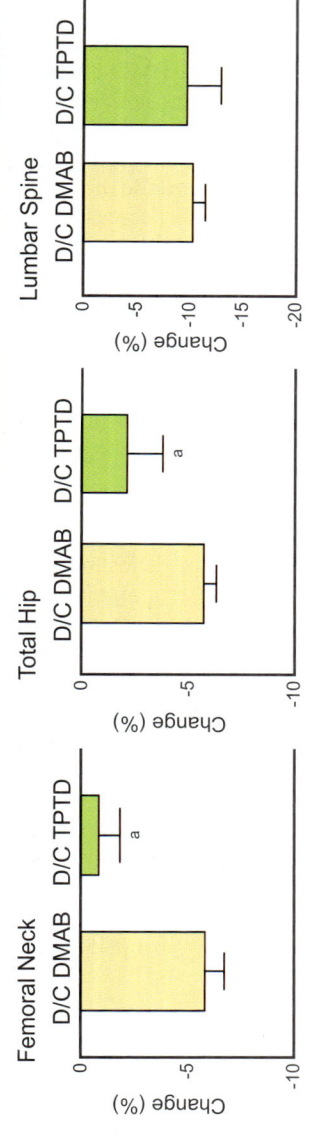

Key: D/C, discontinued; DMAB, denosumab; TPTD, teriparatide.

[a] *P*<0.05 vs D/C TPTD.

Adapted from Leder BZ, et al. *Bone*. 2017;98:54-58.

- All patients should receive calcium 1000 mg daily and at least 400 IU vitamin D daily.
- If a dose is missed, administer the injection as soon as the patient is available. Thereafter, schedule injections every 6 months from the date of the last injection.

Calcitonin

Calcitonin is a polypeptide hormone produced by the parafollicular C cells of the thyroid.

Calcitonin has antiosteoclastic activity:
- Osteoclasts have receptors that bind calcitonin
- Calcitonin inhibits osteoclasts by:
  - Interfering with osteoclast brush borders
  - Inhibiting cytoplasmic motility
  - Decreasing the rate of osteoclast formation.

■ **Efficacy, Side Effects and Dosage, and Administration**

In clinical practice, the most commonly used calcitonin is derived from salmon. Other preparations are derived from human, pig, and an analog of eel calcitonin.

Salmon calcitonin (SCT) is administered either:
- Parenterally, by:
  - IM injection
  - SC injection
- Intranasally.

Available SCT products and their dosing are listed in **Table 9.1**.

Parenteral SCT is indicated for *treatment* of postmenopausal osteoporosis. Some clinically relevant facts include:
- Acts essentially identical to mammalian calcitonins, but its potency and duration of action are greater.
- The majority of randomized, placebo-controlled studies demonstrate greater bone density in

calcitonin-treated patients as early as 3 months after initiation of therapy, with persistence for up to 3 years

- May relieve pain following acute osteoporotic vertebral fractures (short-term therapy)[104]
- Side effects include anorexia, nausea, vomiting, metallic taste, diarrhea, flushing, rash, and pruritus.

Intranasal SCT, which is indicated for the *treatment* of osteoporosis in women who are >5 years postmenopause with low bone mass, has the following characteristics:

- Clinical and biologic effects similar to those of the IM version
- Mean bioavailability of the nasal spray approximately 3% of that of injectable calcitonin in normal subjects
- Significant increases in lumbar vertebral BMD as early as 6 months, with persistence up to 2 years. No effects on cortical bone of forearm or hip demonstrated
- Evidence for fracture prevention is limited. In a randomized placebo-controlled study (PROOF study) in postmenopausal women with osteoporosis, 200 IU intranasal SCT reduced the rate of vertebral fractures by 30% in comparison with placebo.[105] No significant reduction in peripheral fractures was noted. There was also no consistent effect on bone markers and BMD. Doses of 100 and 400 IU had no effect (no dose response was seen).
- Tolerance better than with the parenteral route of administration
- Rhinitis, epistaxis, and sinusitis have occurred in 12%, 3.5%, and 2.3% of patients, respectively.
- An oral calcitonin preparation may be linked to prostate cancer causing European regulatory authorities to modify the label for calcitonin.[106]

- **Dosage and Administration**

Intranasal calcitonin is approved for 200 IU daily alternating nostrils

Subcutaneous or intramuscular calcitonin is administered as 100 IU every other day.

Strontium Ranelate

This compound, composed of two atoms of stable strontium combined with organic ranelic acid, is approved in over 100 countries in Europe, Africa, Latin America, Asia, and Australia (but not approved in the United States) for the prevention and treatment of osteoporosis in postmenopausal women. As an alkaline earth element, strontium is similar to calcium in its absorption in the gut, incorporation into bone, and elimination via the kidneys. Strontium is naturally present in trace amounts in bone.

The mechanism of action by which strontium ranelate increases bone strength and reduces fracture risk has not been clearly established. Studies in humans indicate that it has only weak effects on bone remodeling. Changes in bone material properties associated with incorporation of strontium into bone mineral may be implicated in its therapeutic effects and may result in a partial artifactual increase in its efficacy.

- **Efficacy**

Two large, randomized, placebo-controlled trials assessed the fracture prevention efficacy of strontium ranelate 2 g/day. In the Spinal Osteoporosis Therapeutic Intervention (SOTI) trial the risk of new vertebral fractures was reduced significantly by 49% in the first year of strontium ranelate treatment and 41% during the 3-year period.[107-109] Strontium ranelate also increased BMD at month 36 by 14.4% at the lumbar spine and 8.3% at the femoral neck.

In the Treatment of Peripheral Osteoporosis (TROPOS) trial after 3 years, strontium ranelate treatment significantly reduced the RR by 16% for all nonvertebral fractures, and by 19% for major fragility fractures compared with the placebo group.[110,111] Among women at high risk of hip fracture (age ≥74 years and femoral neck BMD T score ≤-2.4), the RRR for hip fracture was significant at 36%. In a subgroup, the RR of vertebral fractures was significantly reduced by 39% over 3 years and by 45% during the first year of treatment. In patients with at least one prevalent vertebral fracture, the risk of a new vertebral fracture was reduced significantly by 32% over 3 years. In addition, strontium ranelate significantly increased BMD by 8.2% (femoral neck) and 9.8% (total hip) at 3 years.

A pooling of data from the SOTI and TROPOS trials found that there was a significant reduction in the risk of vertebral, nonvertebral, and clinical (symptomatic vertebral and nonvertebral) fractures within 1 year and at the end of 3 years in these elderly patients.[109]

In an open-label extension study pooling data from SOTI and TROPOS, lumbar BMD increased significantly for the 10-year period.[112] There appeared to be sustained efficacy with regard to vertebral and nonvertebral fractures over 10 years.

Although a number of nonprescription products containing other strontium compounds (eg, strontium carbonate, strontium citrate) are widely available in the United States and other countries, there are no clinical data on the efficacy of such products for the prevention or treatment of osteoporosis.

■ Side Effects

In the SOTI trial, diarrhea was the most frequently reported adverse event with strontium ranelate with a higher frequency than in the placebo group (6.1% vs 3.6%).[108] In the TROPOS study, the incidence of nausea (7.2% vs 4.4%), diarrhea (6.7% vs 5.0%), headaches (3.4% vs 2.4%), and dermatitis and eczema (5.5% vs 4.1%) were more frequent in the strontium ranelate group.[111] However, the differences in the frequencies of some of these adverse events (nausea in SOTI and diarrhea and nausea in TROPOS) were no longer observed after 3 months of treatment. Because of an increase in the risk of venous thromboembolic disease (VTE), strontium ranelate is contraindicated in women with current or past VTE and in those who are temporarily or permanently immobilized.

Based on the above, an appropriate choice can be made for a given individual at a specific point in time. Close observation and regular monitoring will ensure optimum care and results.

In a benefit/risk assessment of about 7500 patients from strontium clinical trials, a European agency found an increased risk for adverse cardiovascular events, including MI, in women receiving strontium ranelate compared with those who received placebo. However, there was no increased risk of death. This has led to some labeling changes and proposed restrictions.[113]

■ **Dosage and Administration**

The recommended dosing of strontium ranelate is 2 g orally per day.

Postmenopausal Hormone Replacement Therapy

The use of hormone replacement therapy in perimenopausal and postmenopausal women underwent a dramatic shift following the publication of the results of the Heart and Estrogen/Progestin Replacement Study (HERS) and the WHI trials (**Figure 9.15**).[114,115] As a result, although HT is effective in reducing vertebral, nonvertebral, and hip fracture, it is rarely used solely for this indication and is no longer regarded as a first-line option for prevention of osteoporotic fractures.

Side effects of HT in postmenopausal women include increased risk of breast cancer, stroke, and venous thromboembolism. In addition, there is evidence for an increase in the risk of coronary heart disease in older postmenopausal women and some studies have shown increased risk of ovarian cancer.[114,115] Particularly in healthy younger postmenopausal women,

FIGURE 9.15 — Results of the WHI Showing Comparative Risks and Benefits of Combined Estrogen and Progestin Compared With Placebo

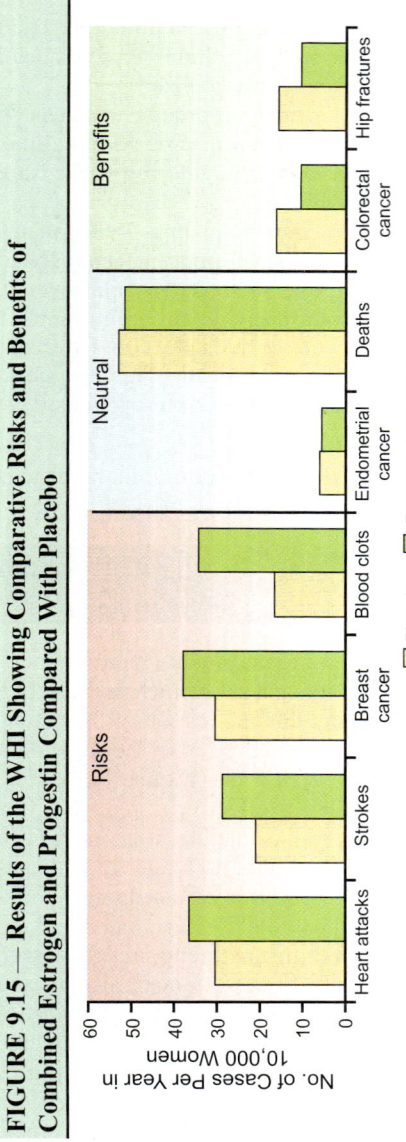

Due to the increased risk of breast cancer and adverse global index, this study was prematurely terminated by the independent data and safety monitoring board.

Adapted from Rossouw JE, et al. *JAMA.* 2002;288(3):321-333.

the absolute risk of developing these conditions is low but rises with increasing age. Use of HT for management of osteoporosis can be summarized as suggested by the National Osteoporosis Society of the UK:

- The decision to take HT must be based on full consultation between a woman and her clinician to ensure that she fully understands the risks and benefits involved with treatment, and its use should be reviewed regularly to account for any change in balance of benefits and risks.
- HT is an effective treatment for menopausal symptoms and for prevention of fractures at both hip and spine for women <60 years of age—it is not appropriate for osteoporosis treatment in women over age 60.
- HT should be recommended for women who have experienced an early menopause at least until the normal age of the menopause (around 50 years of age). This will help reduce bone loss and to avoid the symptoms and other complications of prolonged estrogen deficiency.
- For postmenopausal women below the age of 60 without risk factors for breast cancer, heart disease stroke, or venous thromboembolism, the risks associated with HT are low. For these women, HT can be considered as a treatment for osteoporosis, providing that the beneficial effects on fracture risk reduction outweigh any adverse risks for that individual.
- In women up to the age of 60, who are using HT for relief of menopausal symptoms, it is accepted that the HT benefit normally exceeds risk irrespective of the potential bone effect, which will be an additional benefit.

Parathyroid Hormone Analogues

■ Biologic Basis for Anabolic Effect

Persistent and excessive secretion of PTH (as in both primary and secondary hyperparathyroidism) is associated with bone loss, especially in cortical bone.

Intermittent PTH has a net anabolic effect since there is also a lesser increase in bone resorption (ie, an anabolic window). Animal studies show increases in the mechanical strength of trabecular and cortical bone by stimulation of new bone formation at the periosteal (outer) and endosteal (inner) bone surfaces.[116,117]

The net result is:
- Thickening of the cortices
- Increasing the number and connectivity of the trabeculae.

Mechanisms of PTH action include the following:
- Stimulation on the cells of osteoblastic lineage of the PTH-1 receptor, which is shared by both PTH and PTH-related peptide (PTHrP), thus known as the PTH–PTHrP receptor.
- Amplification of the number of osteoblasts in two ways:
  - Stimulation of cell replication
  - Inhibition of osteoblast apoptosis
- Induction of growth factors
- Inhibition of sclerostin production by osteocytes
- Increasing the cytokine RANKL and the osteoblastic modulation of osteoclast activity.

PTH is an 84-amino acid peptide with its biologic activity located in amino acids 1 through 34. Two recombinant forms of human PTH have been developed consisting of either the 1-34 segment (teriparatide, rhPTH[1-34]) or the complete peptide segment (parathyroid hormone, rhPTH[1-84]); however, only rhPTH(1-34) is approved for the treatment of osteoporosis in the United States. The full-length peptide segment is indicated as an adjunct to calcium and vitamin D to control hypocalcemia in patients with hypoparathyroidism. A human parathyroid hormone related peptide (abaloparatide, PTHrP[1-34]) has also been approved for the treatment of osteoporosis.

■ **Teriparatide (rhPTH[1-34])**

Teriparatide, a recombinant 1-34 amino acid fragment of PTH, is indicated for:

- Treatment of postmenopausal women with osteoporosis at high risk for fracture,
- Increase of bone mass in men with primary or hypogonadal osteoporosis at high risk for fracture, and
- Treatment of men and women with osteoporosis associated with sustained systemic glucocorticoid therapy at high risk for fracture.

Efficacy and safety of teriparatide have been assessed in prospective studies for a period of only 2 years and there may be a limited anabolic window. Further, studies in Fisher rats (not confirmed in primates) demonstrated osteosarcoma leading to an FDA blackbox warning. Thus, the duration of treatment is recommended for only a 2-year interval. When use of teriparatide is stopped, however, a decline in BMD is evident in the following year, although fracture reduction may persist for 1 or 2 years. Bone loss is prevented and, in some cases, there is an increase in BMD when administration of an antiresorptive agent follows teriparatide therapy.[118,119]

Of note, there have been early experiences suggesting efficacy of using PTH even more intermittently than once a day, but alternate modes of administration are not currently widely recommended.[120]

The effect of teriparatide on fracture risk was evaluated in the Fracture Prevention Trial. New vertebral fractures occurred in 14% of the women in the placebo group and in 5% and 4%, respectively, of the women receiving either 20 mcg or 40 mcg teriparatide (**Figure 9.16**).[121] Lumbar spine BMD increased by 13.7% (PTH 40 mcg), 9.7% (PTH 20 mcg), and 1.1% (placebo). Teriparatide (both doses) reduced the risk of new nonvertebral fractures by about 35%. The increases in BMD are shown in **Table 9.4**.

Most side effects reported in association with teriparatide in clinical trials were mild and included nausea,

FIGURE 9.16 — Fracture Prevention Trial: Teriparatide Effect on Vertebral Fractures

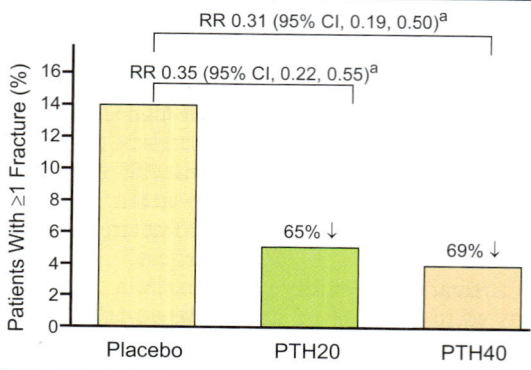

RR 0.31 (95% CI, 0.19, 0.50)[a]

RR 0.35 (95% CI, 0.22, 0.55)[a]

[a] New vertebral fractures occurred in 14%, 5%, and 4% of the PTH 40-mcg, PTH 20-mcg, and placebo groups, respectively. Compared with placebo, PTH treatment reduced the risk of one or more new vertebral fractures by 65% (PTH 20 mcg) and 69% (PTH 40 mcg). $P<0.001$.

Neer RM, et al. *N Engl J Med*. 2001;344(19):1434-1441.

TABLE 9.4 — Fracture Prevention Trial: Percent Changes From Baseline in BMD With Teriparatide

	Placebo	Teriparatide (*P* Value)[a]	
		20 mcg	40 mcg
Lumbar spine	1.1	9.7 (0.001)	13.7 (0.001)
Femoral neck	-0.7	2.8 (0.001)	5.1 (0.001)
Trochanter	-0.2	3.5 (0.001)	4.4 (0.001)
Total hip	-1.0	2.6 (0.001)	3.6 (0.001)

[a] Compared with placebo.

Neer RM, et al. *N Engl J Med*. 2001;344:1434-1441.

dizziness, and leg cramps. During clinical trials, early discontinuation due to adverse events occurred in 5.6% of patients assigned to placebo and 7.1% of patients taking teriparatide. Although there was an increased incidence of osteosarcoma in preclinical studies in rats, there have been no reports of osteosarcoma in human trials. Postmarketing surveillance demonstrates extremely rare cases of osteosarcoma in numbers that mirror the background rate in the general population. Nonetheless, the labeling for teriparatide contains a black box warning about osteosarcoma risk. Due to the small risk of osteosarcoma in patients with Paget's disease, teriparatide should not be prescribed to this group of patients. In addition, teriparatide should not be prescribed in patients with pre-existing hypercalcemia, bone metastases or a history of skeletal malignancies, metabolic bone diseases other than osteoporosis, or pediatric or young adult patients with open epiphyses.

The recommended dose is 20 mcg per day injected subcutaneously in the thigh or abdominal wall. Teriparatide should be administered initially under circumstances in which the patient can sit or lie down if symptoms of orthostatic hypotension occur.

■ **Abaloparatide (PTHrP[1-34])**

Abaloparatide, a synthetic 34 amino acid peptide, is an analog of human parathyroid hormone-related peptide (PTHrP[1-34]), having 76% homology with its human counterpart.[122] It acts as an agonist at the PTH1 receptor, having an anabolic effect on bone, demonstrated through increases in BMD and BMC. It is indicated for the treatment of postmenopausal women with osteoporosis at high risk for fracture defined as a history of osteoporotic fracture, multiple risk factors for fracture, or patients who have failed or are intolerant to other available osteoporosis therapy.

Like teriparatide, abaloparatide has a boxed warning for osteosarcoma since subcutaneous administration caused a dose-dependent increase in the incidence of osteosarcoma in male and female rats. It is unknown whether it causes osteosarcoma in humans, but the cumulative use of abaloparatide and parathyroid hormone analogs (eg, teriparatide) for more than 2 years during a patient's lifetime is not recommended.

The efficacy of abaloparatide for the treatment of postmenopausal osteoporosis was evaluated in two clinical trials: ACTIVE and ACTIVExtend.[123,124] The cumulative 25-month efficacy dataset included 18 months of exposure to abaloparatide 80 mcg or placebo in the ACTIVE trial, 1 month of no treatment, followed by 6 months of alendronate therapy in the ACTIVExtend extension study. At 18 months, new vertebral fractures occurred in 0.6% of women in the abaloparatide group and in 4.2% of women receiving placebo (P <0.0001), and remained similarly and significantly lower in the abaloparatide treatment group at 25 months (**Figure 9.17**). Significant greater reductions in the incidence of nonvertebral fractures were also observed at 18 months in the abaloparatide group (2.7%) compared to the placebo group (4.7%) (**Figure 9.18**). At 25 months, the cumulative incidence of nonvertebral fractures was 2.7% for women who previously received abaloparatide compared to 5.6% for women who had received placebo. The effects of abaloparatide on the risk of vertebral and nonvertebral fractures were consistent regardless of age, years since menopause, presence or absence of prior fracture, and BMD at baseline. Treatment with abaloparatide for 18 months also resulted in significantly greater increases in BMD compared to placebo for lumbar spine, total hip, and femoral neck (P <0.0001 each), with similar results at month 25.

The most common adverse events experienced by postmenopausal women treated with abaloparatide were hypercalciuria (11%), dizziness (10%), nausea (8%), and headache (8%). The proportion of patients who discontinued the study drug due to adverse events was 10% in the abaloparatide group and 6% in the placebo group. Abaloparatide is not recommended in patients at increased risk of osteosarcoma, including those with Paget's disease of bone, unexplained elevations of alkaline phosphatase, open epiphyses, bone metastases or skeletal malignancies, hereditary disorders predisposing to osteosarcoma, or prior external beam or implant radiation therapy involving the skeleton. Additionally, it is not recommended in patients with pre-existing hypercalcemia, or in patients who have an underlying hypercalcemic disorder.

The recommended dosage of abaloparatide is 80 mcg subcutaneously once daily, administered at approximately the same time each day into the periumbilical region of the abdomen. Patients should receive supplemental calcium and vitamin D if dietary intake is inadequate. As with teriparatide, orthostatic hypotension may occur following administration of abaloparatide. For this reason, for the first several doses, abaloparatide should be administered where the patient can sit or lie down if necessary.

■ **PTH in Combination or Following Antiresorptive Therapy**

When PTH is given concurrently with daily anti-resorptive therapy in patients naive to both drugs, there is an attenuation in BMD increases compared with PTH alone.[125] (**Figure 9.19**) Biochemical markers of bone formation are also suppressed by this combination approach. In contrast, when PTH is administered in combination with a potent IV bisphosphonate, there is a synergistic effect on BMD (**Figure 9.20**).[126] In patients who are longer-term users of bisphosphonates, PTH effects do not appear to attenuate BMD as much.

A secondary analysis of EUROFORS in women treated with open-label teriparatide who had previous treatment with an antiresorptive agent—alendronate, risedronate, etidronate, and non-bisphosphonate (for at least 12 months), relative to baseline, there were significant increases in lumbar spine BMD at all time points in each subgroup.[127] Notably, there were significantly greater lumbar spine BMD increases at all time points in women previously treated with etidronate compared with women previously treated with alendronate and risedronate, and at 18 and 24 months compared with

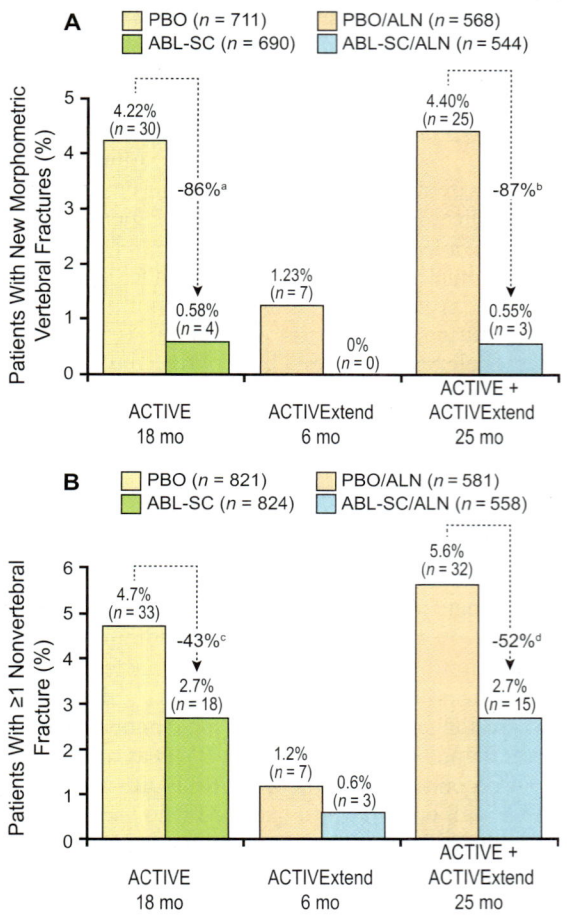

Continued

Key: ABL-SC, subcutaneous abaloparatide; ALN, alendronate; PBO, placebo.

[a] *P*<0.001 vs PBO.
[b] Relative risk, 0.13; 95% CI, 0.04-0.41; *P*<0.001 vs PBO/ALN.
[c] *P*<0.05 vs PBO.
[d] Hazard ratio, 0.48; 95% CI, 0.26-0.89; log-rank *P*=0.02 vs PBO/ALN.

Adapted from Cosman F, et al. *Mayo Clin Proc*. 2017;92(2):200-210.

FIGURE 9.18 — ACTIVE Trial: Kaplan–Meier Curve of Time to First Incident Nonvertebral Fractures by Treatment Group (ITT Population)

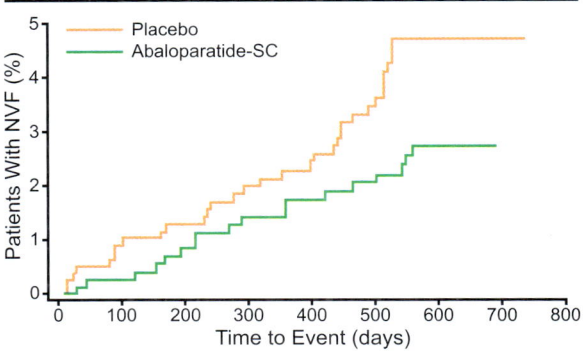

Key: ITT, intention-to-treat; NVF, nonvertebral fracture.
Log-rank *P*-value:
• Abaloparatide-SC vs placebo: 0.0489

Modified from Miller PD. *JAMA*. 2016;316(7):722-733.

9

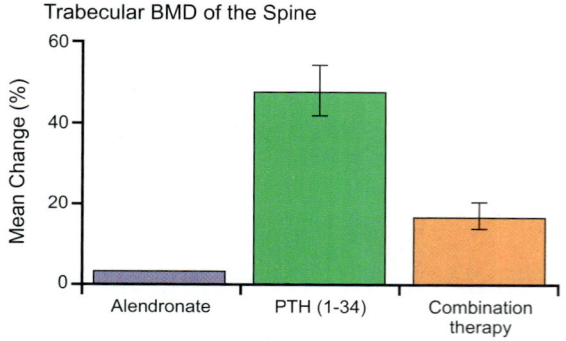

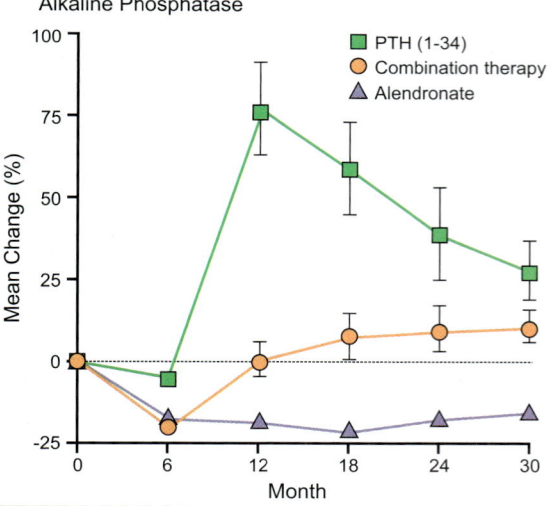

Finkelstein JS, et al. *N Engl J Med.* 2003;349(13): 1216-1226.

FIGURE 9.20 — Synergistic Effects on Lumbar Spine BMD of a Combination of Zoledronic Acid and Teriparatide Compared With Either Agent Alone

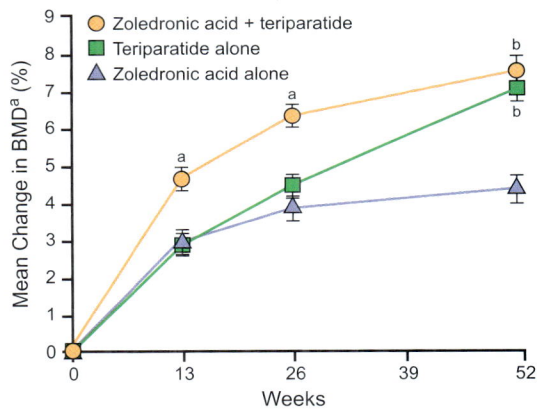

[a] $P<0.0001$ vs teriparatide alone and vs zoledronic acid alone.

[b] $P<0.0001$ vs zoledronic acid alone.

Cosman F et al. *J Bone Miner Res*. 2011;26(3):503-511.

women previously treated with non-bisphosphonates. Changes in BMD and biochemical markers of bone formation indicated that treatment with teriparatide induces positive effects on bone mass and osteoblast function regardless of previous long-term exposure to antiresorptive therapies in postmenopausal women with established osteoporosis, although there is some blunting of the BMD response with more potent antiresorptive agents. Duration of antiresorptive therapy and lag time between stopping previous therapy and starting teriparatide did not affect the BMD response at any skeletal site.

■ PTH and Glucocorticoid-Induced Osteoporosis

Women and men who had received ≥5 mg/day of prednisone for ≥3 months preceding screening for the trial had increases from baseline in lumbar spine, total hip, and femoral neck BMD were significantly greater in patients taking teriparatide than in those receiving daily alendronate group.[128,129] Similarly, there were significant median percent increases from baseline in all bone formation markets after 1, 6, 18, and 36 months with teriparatide compared with alendronate. A significantly greater number of vertebral fractures occurred in the alendronate group than in the teriparatide group over the same period, but there were no significant differences in nonvertebral fractures. Teriparatide was generally well tolerated.

■ **PTH and Trabecular Connectivity**

Lattice distribution in trabecular bone influences bone strength independently of trabecular bone volume.

Current antiresorptive therapies cannot reconnect disrupted trabecular plates. A histomorphometric study in iliac crest biopsies before and after treatment with 40 mcg of rhPTH(1-34), revealed the following[130]:

- Anabolic effect on cancellous bone volume
- Anabolic effect on cortical bone
- Increased connectivity between trabecular struts.

This study provides documentation of a structural basis for the reduction of osteoporotic fractures in women (**Figure 9.21**).

Long-term Osteoporosis Treatment— Current Perspective

For most anti-osteoporosis agents, the evidence for antifracture efficacy beyond 5 years of treatment is weak or insufficient to make evaluations beyond that time. Among the bisphosphonates, there is established fracture efficacy up to 3 years, and up to 4 or 5 years for alendronate and risedronate. Stabilized bone mass or sustained increases in BMD are evident beyond 5 years. The safety of bisphosphonates does not appear

FIGURE 9.21 — PTH Increased Trabecular Connectivity and Cortical Wall Thickness

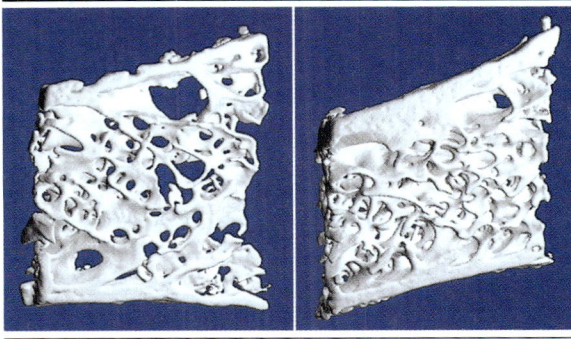

In these scanning electron micrographs of a 64-year-old woman, connectivity density and cortex thickness are shown to have increased after PTH therapy. Before PTH therapy *(left)* connectivity density was $2.9/mm^3$ and cortex thickness was 0.32 mm. Following PTH therapy *(right)* these measurements were shown to have improved to $4.6/mm^3$ and 0.42 mm, respectively.

Dempster DW, et al. *J Bone Miner Res*. 2001;16:1846-1853.

to be compromised with time, although there is the association with rare atypical femoral fracture and ONJ, both of which appear to be related to duration of therapy. Given their skeletal retention, sustained benefits in patients with prolonged therapy, and emerging safety concerns, a bisphosphonate "holiday" after 5 years of oral therapy or at least one intravenous infusion of zoledronic acid may be considered. In 8 years of testing, denosumab has demonstrated continued increases in BMD and long-term safety appears satisfactory. However, in contrast to bisphosphonates, a "drug holiday" is not recommended for denosumab, due to the rapid increase in bone remodeling and bone loss accompanying treatment discontinuation that may increase fracture risk. Strontium ranelate has demonstrated fracture efficacy and provides sustained increases in BMD over 10 years. Its long-term safety record has recently been questioned with regard to cardiovascular events. PTH is the only currently available bone-stimulating agent. It results in significant increases in trabecular BMD and a reduction in vertebral fracture risk, albeit at a higher cost and inconvenience than some of the other agents currently available. Its use is generally limited to a single 18- to 24-month duration of therapy.

REFERENCES

1. Kanis JA, Burlet N, Cooper C, et al. European guidance for the diagnosis and management of osteoporosis in postmenopausal women. *Osteoporos Int*. 2008;19(4):399-428.

2. Sambrook P, Cooper C. Osteoporosis. *Lancet*. 2006;367(9527): 2010-2018.

3. Diez-Perez A. Bisphosphonates. *Maturitas*. 2002;43(suppl 1): S19-S26.

4. Plotkin LI, Weinstein RS, Parfitt AM, et al. Prevention of osteocyte and osteoblast apoptosis by bisphosphonates and calcitonin. *J Clin Invest*. 1999;104(10):1363-1374.

5. Black DM, Thompson DE, Bauer DC, et al. Fracture risk reduction with alendronate in women with osteoporosis: the Fracture Intervention Trial. FIT Research Group. *J Clin Endocrinol Metab*. 2000;85(11):4118-4124.

6. Pols HA, Felsenberg D, Hanley DA, et al. Multinational, placebo-controlled, randomized trial of the effects of alendronate on bone density and fracture risk in postmenopausal women with low bone mass: results of the FOSIT study. Fosamax International Trial Study Group. *Osteoporos Int*. 1999;9(5):461-468.

7. Hochberg MC, Thompson DE, Black DM, et al. Effect of alendronate on the age-specific incidence of symptomatic osteoporotic fractures. *J Bone Miner Res*. 2005;20(6):971-976.

8. Luckey MM, Gilchrist N, Bone HG, et al. Therapeutic equivalence of alendronate 35 milligrams once weekly and 5 milligrams daily in the prevention of postmenopausal osteoporosis. *Obstet Gynecol*. 2003;101(4):711-721.

9. Rizzoli R, Greenspan SL, Bone G, 3rd, et al. Two-year results of once-weekly administration of alendronate 70 mg for the treatment of postmenopausal osteoporosis. *J Bone Miner Res*. 2002;17(11):1988-1996.

10. Schnitzer T, Bone HG, Crepaldi G, et al. Therapeutic equivalence of alendronate 70 mg once-weekly and alendronate 10 mg daily in the treatment of osteoporosis. Alendronate Once-Weekly Study Group. *Aging (Milano)*. 2000;12(1):1-12.

11. Bonnick S, Saag KG, Kiel DP, et al. Comparison of weekly treatment of postmenopausal osteoporosis with alendronate versus risedronate over two years. *J Clin Endocrinol Metab*. 2006;91(7):2631-2637.

12. Reid DM, Hosking D, Kendler D, et al. Alendronic acid produces greater effects than risedronic acid on bone density and turnover in postmenopausal women with osteoporosis : results of FACTS -international. *Clin Drug Investig*. 2006;26(2):63-74.

13. Rosen CJ, Hochberg MC, Bonnick SL, et al. Treatment with once-weekly alendronate 70 mg compared with once-weekly risedronate 35 mg in women with postmenopausal osteoporosis: a randomized double-blind study. *J Bone Miner Res*. 2005;20(1):141-151.

14. Black DM, Schwartz AV, Ensrud KE, et al. Effects of continuing or stopping alendronate after 5 years of treatment: the Fracture Intervention Trial Long-term Extension (FLEX): a randomized trial. *JAMA*. 2006;296(24):2927-2938.

15. Schwartz AV, Bauer DC, Cummings SR, et al. Efficacy of continued alendronate for fractures in women with and without prevalent vertebral fracture: the FLEX trial. *J Bone Miner Res*. 2010;25(5):976-982.

16. Adachi JD, Saag KG, Delmas PD, et al. Two-year effects of alendronate on bone mineral density and vertebral fracture in patients receiving glucocorticoids: a randomized, double-blind, placebo-controlled extension trial. *Arthritis Rheum*. 2001;44(1):202-211.

17. Saag KG, Emkey R, Schnitzer TJ, et al. Alendronate for the prevention and treatment of glucocorticoid-induced osteoporosis. Glucocorticoid-Induced Osteoporosis Intervention Study Group. *N Engl J Med*. 1998;339(5):292-299.

18. Kanis JA, Stevenson M, McCloskey EV, et al. Glucocorticoid-induced osteoporosis: a systematic review and cost-utility analysis. *Health Technol Assess*. 2007;11(7):iii-iv, ix-xi, 1-231.

19. Borah B, Dufresne TE, Chmielewski PA, et al. Risedronate preserves trabecular architecture and increases bone strength in vertebra of ovariectomized minipigs as measured by three-dimensional microcomputed tomography. *J Bone Miner Res*. 2002;17(7):1139-1147.

20. Borah B, Dufresne TE, Ritman EL, et al. Long-term risedronate treatment normalizes mineralization and continues to preserve

trabecular architecture: sequential triple biopsy studies with micro-computed tomography. *Bone*. 2006;39(2):345-352.

21. Hooper MJ, Ebeling PR, Roberts AP, et al. Risedronate prevents bone loss in early postmenopausal women: a prospective randomized, placebo-controlled trial. *Climacteric*. 2005;8(3): 251-262.

22. Harris ST, Watts NB, Genant HK, et al. Effects of risedronate treatment on vertebral and nonvertebral fractures in women with postmenopausal osteoporosis: a randomized controlled trial. Vertebral Efficacy With Risedronate Therapy (VERT) Study Group. *JAMA*. 1999;282(14):1344-1352.

23. Reginster J, Minne HW, Sorensen OH, et al. Randomized trial of the effects of risedronate on vertebral fractures in women with established postmenopausal osteoporosis. Vertebral Efficacy with Risedronate Therapy (VERT) Study Group. *Osteoporos Int*. 2000;11(1):83-91.

24. Eastell R, Barton I, Hannon RA, et al. Relationship of early changes in bone resorption to the reduction in fracture risk with risedronate. *J Bone Miner Res*. 2003;18(6):1051-1056.

25. Mellstrom DD, Sorensen OH, Goemaere S, et al. Seven years of treatment with risedronate in women with postmenopausal osteoporosis. *Calcif Tissue Int*. 2004;75(6):462-468.

26. Sorensen OH, Crawford GM, Mulder H, et al. Long-term efficacy of risedronate: a 5-year placebo-controlled clinical experience. *Bone*. 2003;32(2):120-126.

27. McClung MR, Geusens P, Miller PD, et al. Effect of risedronate on the risk of hip fracture in elderly women. Hip Intervention Program Study Group. *N Engl J Med*. 2001;344(5):333-340.

28. Brown JP, Kendler DL, McClung MR, et al. The efficacy and tolerability of risedronate once a week for the treatment of postmenopausal osteoporosis. *Calcif Tissue Int*. 2002;71(2):103-111.

29. Delmas PD, Benhamou CL, Man Z, et al. Monthly dosing of 75 mg risedronate on 2 consecutive days a month: efficacy and safety results. *Osteoporos Int*. 2008;19(7):1039-1045.

30. Reid DM, Hughes RA, Laan RF, et al. Efficacy and safety of daily risedronate in the treatment of corticosteroid-induced osteoporosis in men and women: a randomized trial. European Corticosteroid-Induced Osteoporosis Treatment Study. *J Bone Miner Res*. 2000;15(6):1006-1013.

31. Cohen S, Levy RM, Keller M, et al. Risedronate therapy prevents corticosteroid-induced bone loss: a twelve-month, multicenter, randomized, double-blind, placebo-controlled, parallel-group study. *Arthritis Rheum*. 1999;42(11):2309-2318.

32. Wallach S, Cohen S, Reid DM, et al. Effects of risedronate treatment on bone density and vertebral fracture in patients on corticosteroid therapy. *Calcif Tissue Int.* 2000;67(4):277-285.

33. Barrett J, Worth E, Bauss F, et al. Ibandronate: a clinical pharmacological and pharmacokinetic update. *J Clin Pharmacol.* 2004;44(9):951-965.

34. Riis BJ, Ise J, von Stein T, et al. Ibandronate: a comparison of oral daily dosing versus intermittent dosing in postmenopausal osteoporosis. *J Bone Miner Res.* 2001;16(10):1871-1878.

35. Delmas PD, Adami S, Strugala C, et al. Intravenous ibandronate injections in postmenopausal women with osteoporosis: one-year results from the dosing intravenous administration study. *Arthritis Rheum.* 2006;54(6):1838-1846.

36. Eisman JA, Civitelli R, Adami S, et al. Efficacy and tolerability of intravenous ibandronate injections in postmenopausal osteoporosis: 2-year results from the DIVA study. *J Rheumatol.* 2008;35(3):488-497.

37. Lewiecki EM, Keaveny TM, Kopperdahl DL, et al. Once-monthly oral ibandronate improves biomechanical determinants of bone strength in women with postmenopausal osteoporosis. *J Clin Endocrinol Metab.* 2009;94(1):171-180.

38. Pyon EY. Once-monthly ibandronate for postmenopausal osteoporosis: review of a new dosing regimen. *Clin Ther.* 2006; 28(4):475-490.

39. Chesnut IC, Skag A, Christiansen C, et al. Effects of oral ibandronate administered daily or intermittently on fracture risk in postmenopausal osteoporosis. *J Bone Miner Res.* 2004;19(8): 1241-1249.

40. Miller PD, McClung MR, Macovei L, et al. Monthly oral ibandronate therapy in postmenopausal osteoporosis: 1-year results from the MOBILE study. *J Bone Miner Res.* 2005;20(8):1315-1322.

41. Reginster JY, Adami S, Lakatos P, et al. Efficacy and tolerability of once-monthly oral ibandronate in postmenopausal osteoporosis: 2 year results from the MOBILE study. *Ann Rheum Dis.* 2006;65(5):654-661.

42. McClung MR, Wasnich RD, Recker R, et al. Oral daily ibandronate prevents bone loss in early postmenopausal women without osteoporosis. *J Bone Miner Res.* 2004;19(1):11-18.

43. Stakkestad JA, Benevolenskaya LI, Stepan JJ, et al. Intravenous ibandronate injections given every three months: a new treatment option to prevent bone loss in postmenopausal women. *Ann Rheum Dis.* 2003;62(10):969-975.

44. Adami S, Felsenberg D, Christiansen C, et al. Efficacy and safety of ibandronate given by intravenous injection once every 3 months. *Bone*. 2004;34(5):881-889.

45. Black DM, Delmas PD, Eastell R, et al. Once-yearly zoledronic acid for treatment of postmenopausal osteoporosis. *N Engl J Med*. 2007;356(18):1809-1822.

46. Compston J. Treatments for osteoporosis - looking beyond the HORIZON. *N Engl J Med*. 2007;356(18):1878-1880.

47. Colon-Emeric CS, Caminis J, Suh TT, et al. The HORIZON Recurrent Fracture Trial: design of a clinical trial in the prevention of subsequent fractures after low trauma hip fracture repair. *Curr Med Res Opin*. 2004;20(6):903-910.

48. Lyles KW, Colon-Emeric CS, Magaziner JS, et al. Zoledronic acid and clinical fractures and mortality after hip fracture. *N Engl J Med*. 2007;357(18):1799-1809.

49. Cauley JA, Black D, Boonen S, et al. Once-yearly zoledronic acid and days of disability, bed rest, and back pain: randomized, controlled HORIZON Pivotal Fracture Trial. *J Bone Miner Res*. 2011;26(5):984-992.

50. Black DM, Reid IR, Boonen S, et al. The effect of 3 versus 6 years of zoledronic acid treatment of osteoporosis: a randomized extension to the HORIZON-Pivotal Fracture Trial (PFT). *J Bone Miner Res*. 2012;27(2):243-254.

51. Reid IR, Black DM, Eastell R, et al. Reduction in the risk of clinical fractures after a single dose of zoledronic Acid 5 milligrams. *J Clin Endocrinol Metab*. 2013;98(2):557-563.

52. Donahue JG, Chan KA, Andrade SE, et al. Gastric and duodenal safety of daily alendronate. *Arch Intern Med*. 2002;162(8): 936-942.

53. Lanza F, Sahba B, Schwartz H, et al. The upper GI safety and tolerability of oral alendronate at a dose of 70 milligrams once weekly: a placebo-controlled endoscopy study. *Am J Gastroenterol*. 2002;97(1):58-64.

54. Cardwell CR, Abnet CC, Cantwell MM, et al. Exposure to oral bisphosphonates and risk of esophageal cancer. *JAMA*. 2010;304(6):657-663.

55. Green J, Czanner G, Reeves G, et al. Oral bisphosphonates and risk of cancer of oesophagus, stomach, and colorectum: case-control analysis within a UK primary care cohort. *BMJ*. 2010;341:c4444.

56. Hoff AO, Toth BB, Altundag K, et al. Frequency and risk factors associated with osteonecrosis of the jaw in cancer patients treated with intravenous bisphosphonates. *J Bone Miner Res*. 2008;23(6):826-836.

57. Bilezikian JP. Osteonecrosis of the jaw–do bisphosphonates pose a risk? *N Engl J Med.* 2006;355(22):2278-2281.

58. Woo SB, Hellstein JW, Kalmar JR. Narrative [corrected] review: bisphosphonates and osteonecrosis of the jaws. *Ann Intern Med.* 2006;144(10):753-761.

59. Hellstein JW, Adler RA, Edwards B, et al. Managing the care of patients receiving antiresorptive therapy for prevention and treatment of osteoporosis: executive summary of recommendations from the American Dental Association Council on Scientific Affairs. *J Am Dent Assoc.* 2011;142(11):1243-1251.

60. Park-Wyllie LY, Mamdani MM, Juurlink DN, et al. Bisphosphonate use and the risk of subtrochanteric or femoral shaft fractures in older women. *JAMA.* 2011;305(8):783-789.

61. Schilcher J, Michaelsson K, Aspenberg P. Bisphosphonate use and atypical fractures of the femoral shaft. *N Engl J Med.* 2011;364(18):1728-1737.

62. Whitaker M, Guo J, Kehoe T, et al. Bisphosphonates for osteoporosis–where do we go from here? *N Engl J Med.* 2012;366(22):2048-2051.

63. Shane E, Burr D, Ebeling PR, et al. Atypical subtrochanteric and diaphyseal femoral fractures: report of a task force of the American Society for Bone and Mineral Research. *J Bone Miner Res.* 2010;25(11):2267-2294.

64. Rizzoli R, Akesson K, Bouxsein M, et al. Subtrochanteric fractures after long-term treatment with bisphosphonates: a European Society on Clinical and Economic Aspects of Osteoporosis and Osteoarthritis, and International Osteoporosis Foundation Working Group Report. *Osteoporos Int.* 2011; 22(2):373-390.

65. McClung M, Harris ST, Miller PD, et al. Bisphosphonate therapy for osteoporosis: benefits, risks, and drug holiday. *Am J Med.* 2013;126(1):13-20.

66. Miller PD, Roux C, Boonen S, et al. Safety and efficacy of risedronate in patients with age-related reduced renal function as estimated by the Cockcroft and Gault method: a pooled analysis of nine clinical trials. *J Bone Miner Res.* 2005;20(12):2105-2115.

67. Kim SY, Kim MJ, Cadarette SM, et al. Bisphosphonates and risk of atrial fibrillation: a meta-analysis. *Arthritis Res Ther.* 2010;12(1):R30.

68. Eriksen EF, Lyles KW, Colon-Emeric CS, et al. Antifracture efficacy and reduction of mortality in relation to timing of the first dose of zoledronic acid after hip fracture. *J Bone Miner Res.* 2009;24(7):1308-1313.

9

69. Bobba RS, Beattie K, Parkinson B, et al. Tolerability of different dosing regimens of bisphosphonates for the treatment of osteoporosis and malignant bone disease. *Drug Saf.* 2006;29(12):1133-1152.

70. Marini JC. Do bisphosphonates make children's bones better or brittle? *N Engl J Med.* 2003;349(5):423-426.

71. Draper MW, Flowers DE, Huster WJ, et al. A controlled trial of raloxifene (LY139481) HCl: impact on bone turnover and serum lipid profile in healthy postmenopausal women. *J Bone Miner Res.* 1996;11(6):835-842.

72. Cooper C, Reginster JY, Cortet B, et al. Long-term treatment of osteoporosis in postmenopausal women: a review from the European Society for Clinical and Economic Aspects of Osteoporosis and Osteoarthritis (ESCEO) and the International Osteoporosis Foundation (IOF). *Curr Med Res Opin.* 2012;28(3):475-491.

73. Ettinger B, Black DM, Mitlak BH, et al. Reduction of vertebral fracture risk in postmenopausal women with osteoporosis treated with raloxifene: results from a 3-year randomized clinical trial. Multiple Outcomes of Raloxifene Evaluation (MORE) Investigators. *JAMA.* 1999;282(7):637-645.

74. Johnell O, Kanis JA, Black DM, et al. Associations between baseline risk factors and vertebral fracture risk in the Multiple Outcomes of Raloxifene Evaluation (MORE) Study. *J Bone Miner Res.* 2004;19(5):764-772.

75. Jolly EE, Bjarnason NH, Neven P, et al. Prevention of osteoporosis and uterine effects in postmenopausal women taking raloxifene for 5 years. *Menopause.* 2003;10(4):337-344.

76. Vogel VG, Costantino JP, Wickerham DL, et al. Effects of tamoxifen vs raloxifene on the risk of developing invasive breast cancer and other disease outcomes: the NSABP Study of Tamoxifen and Raloxifene (STAR) P-2 trial. *JAMA.* 2006; 295(23):2727-2741.

77. Siris ES, Harris ST, Eastell R, et al. Skeletal effects of raloxifene after 8 years: results from the continuing outcomes relevant to Evista (CORE) study. *J Bone Miner Res.* 2005;20(9):1514-1524.

78. Yaffe K, Krueger K, Sarkar S, et al. Cognitive function in postmenopausal women treated with raloxifene. *N Engl J Med.* 2001;344(16):1207-1213.

79. Cauley JA, Norton L, Lippman ME, et al. Continued breast cancer risk reduction in postmenopausal women treated with raloxifene: 4-year results from the MORE trial. Multiple

outcomes of raloxifene evaluation. *Breast Cancer Res Treat.* 2001;65(2):125-134.

80. Mosca L, Grady D, Barrett-Connor E, et al. Effect of raloxifene on stroke and venous thromboembolism according to subgroups in postmenopausal women at increased risk of coronary heart disease. *Stroke.* 2009;40(1):147-155.

81. Gallagher JC, Baylink DJ, Freeman R, et al. Prevention of bone loss with tibolone in postmenopausal women: results of two randomized, double-blind, placebo-controlled, dose-finding studies. *J Clin Endocrinol Metab.* 2001;86(10):4717-4726.

82. Bjarnason NH, Bjarnason K, Haarbo J, et al. Tibolone: prevention of bone loss in late postmenopausal women. *J Clin Endocrinol Metab.* 1996;81(7):2419-2422.

83. Rymer J, Robinson J, Fogelman I. Ten years of treatment with tibolone 2.5 mg daily: effects on bone loss in postmenopausal women. *Climacteric.* 2002;5(4):390-398.

84. Roux C, Pelissier C, Fechtenbaum J, et al. Randomized, double-masked, 2-year comparison of tibolone with 17beta-estradiol and norethindrone acetate in preventing postmenopausal bone loss. *Osteoporos Int.* 2002;13(3):241-248.

85. Cummings SR, Ettinger B, Delmas PD, et al. The effects of tibolone in older postmenopausal women. *N Engl J Med.* 2008; 359(7):697-708.

86. Rubin CD. Treatment considerations in the management of age-related osteoporosis. *Am J Med Sci.* 1999;318(3):158-170.

87. Bjarnason NH, Bjarnason K, Haarbo J, et al. Tibolone: influence on markers of cardiovascular disease. *J Clin Endocrinol Metab.* 1997;82(6):1752-1756.

88. Formoso G, Perrone E, Maltoni S, et al. Short and long term effects of tibolone in postmenopausal women. *Cochrane Database Syst Rev.* 2012;2:CD008536.

89. Kenemans P, Bundred NJ, Foidart JM, et al. Safety and efficacy of tibolone in breast-cancer patients with vasomotor symptoms: a double-blind, randomised, non-inferiority trial. *Lancet Oncol.* 2009;10(2):135-146.

90. Cummings SR. LIFT study is discontinued. *BMJ.* 2006;332 (7542):667.

91. McClung MR, Lewiecki EM, Cohen SB, et al. Denosumab in postmenopausal women with low bone mineral density. *N Engl J Med.* 2006;354(8):821-831.

92. Cummings SR, San Martin J, McClung MR, et al. Denosumab for prevention of fractures in postmenopausal women with osteoporosis. *N Engl J Med.* 2009;361(8):756-765.

9

93. Miller PD, Bolognese MA, Lewiecki EM, et al. Effect of denosumab on bone density and turnover in postmenopausal women with low bone mass after long-term continued, discontinued, and restarting of therapy: a randomized blinded phase 2 clinical trial. *Bone*. 2008;43(2):222-229.

94. Miller PD, Wagman RB, Peacock M, et al. Effect of denosumab on bone mineral density and biochemical markers of bone turnover: six-year results of a phase 2 clinical trial. *J Clin Endocrinol Metab*. 2011;96(2):394-402.

95. Boonen S, Adachi JD, Man Z, et al. Treatment with denosumab reduces the incidence of new vertebral and hip fractures in postmenopausal women at high risk. *J Clin Endocrinol Metab*. 2011;96(6):1727-1736.

96. Papapoulos S, Lippuner K, Roux C, et al. The effect of 8 or 5 years of denosumab treatment in postmenopausal women with osteoporosis: results from the FREEDOM Extension study. *Osteoporos Int*. 2015;26(12):2773-2783.

97. Bone HG, Bolognese MA, Yuen CK, et al. Effects of denosumab on bone mineral density and bone turnover in postmenopausal women. *J Clin Endocrinol Metab*. 2008;93(6): 2149-2157.

98. Brown JP, Prince RL, Deal C, et al. Comparison of the effect of denosumab and alendronate on BMD and biochemical markers of bone turnover in postmenopausal women with low bone mass: a randomized, blinded, phase 3 trial. *J Bone Miner Res*. 2009;24(1):153-161.

99. Kendler D, Benhamou C, Brown JP, et al. Effects of Denosumab vs Alendronate on Bone Mineral Density (BMD), Bone Turnover Markers (BTM), and Safety in Women Previously Treated with Alendronate. *J Bone Miner Res*. 2008;23(suppl 1):M395.

100. Tsai JN, Uihlein AV, Lee H, et al. Teriparatide and denosumab, alone or combined, in women with postmenopausal osteoporosis: the DATA study randomised trial. *Lancet*. 2013;382(9886):50-56.

101. Leder BZ, Tsai JN, Uihlein AV, et al. Denosumab and teriparatide transitions in postmenopausal osteoporosis (the DATA-Switch study): extension of a randomised controlled trial. *Lancet*. 2015;386(9999):1147-1155.

102. Leder BZ, Tsai JN, Jiang LA, et al. Importance of prompt antiresorptive therapy in postmenopausal women discontinuing teriparatide or denosumab: The Denosumab and Teriparatide Follow-up study (DATA-Follow-up). *Bone*. 2017;98:54-58.

103. McClung MR. Cancel the denosumab holiday. *Osteoporos Int.* 2016;27(5):1677-1682.

104. Siminoski K, Josse RG. Prevention and management of osteoporosis: consensus statements from the Scientific Advisory Board of the Osteoporosis Society of Canada. 9. Calcitonin in the treatment of osteoporosis. *CMAJ.* 1996;155(7):962-965.

105. Chesnut CH 3rd, Silverman S, Andriano K, et al. A randomized trial of nasal spray salmon calcitonin in postmenopausal women with established osteoporosis: the prevent recurrence of osteoporotic fractures study. PROOF Study Group. *Am J Med.* 2000;109(4):267-276.

106. European Medicines Agency. Questions and answers on the review of calcitonin-containing medicine. European Medicines Agency Web site. http://www.emea.europa.eu/docs/en_GB/document_library/Referrals_document/Calcitonin_31/WC500130149.pdf. Published July 19, 2012. Accessed May 31, 2017.

107. Blake GM, Fogelman I. Long-term effect of strontium ranelate treatment on BMD. *J Bone Miner Res.* 2005;20(11):1901-1904.

108. Meunier PJ, Roux C, Seeman E, et al. The effects of strontium ranelate on the risk of vertebral fracture in women with postmenopausal osteoporosis. *N Engl J Med.* 2004;350(5):459-468.

109. Seeman E, Vellas B, Benhamou C, et al. Strontium ranelate reduces the risk of vertebral and nonvertebral fractures in women eighty years of age and older. *J Bone Miner Res.* 2006; 21(7):1113-1120.

110. Adami S. Protelos: nonvertebral and hip antifracture efficacy in postmenopausal osteoporosis. *Bone.* 2006;38(2 suppl 1):23-27.

111. Reginster JY, Seeman E, De Vernejoul MC, et al. Strontium ranelate reduces the risk of nonvertebral fractures in postmenopausal women with osteoporosis: Treatment of Peripheral Osteoporosis (TROPOS) study. *J Clin Endocrinol Metab.* 2005; 90(5):2816-2822.

112. Reginster JY, Kaufman JM, Goemaere S, et al. Maintenance of antifracture efficacy over 10 years with strontium ranelate in postmenopausal osteoporosis. *Osteoporos Int.* 2012;23(3): 1115-1122.

113. European Medicines Agency. Recommendation to restrict the use of Protelos/Osseor (strontium ranelate). European Medicines Agency Web site. http://www.ema.europa.eu/docs/en_GB/document_library/Press_release/2013/04/WC500142507.pdf. Published April 23, 2013. Accessed May 31, 2017.

9

114. Manson JE, Hsia J, Johnson KC, et al. Estrogen plus progestin and the risk of coronary heart disease. *N Engl J Med*. 2003; 349(6):523-534.

115. Rossouw JE, Anderson GL, Prentice RL, et al. Risks and benefits of estrogen plus progestin in healthy postmenopausal women: principal results From the Women's Health Initiative randomized controlled trial. *JAMA*. 2002;288(3):321-333.

116. Parfitt AM. Parathyroid hormone and periosteal bone expansion. *J Bone Miner Res*. 2002;17(10):1741-1743.

117. Rubin MR, Cosman F, Lindsay R, et al. The anabolic effects of parathyroid hormone. *Osteoporos Int*. 2002;13(4):267-277.

118. Bilezikian JP, Rubin MR. Combination/sequential therapies for anabolic and antiresorptive skeletal agents for osteoporosis. *Curr Osteoporos Rep*. 2006;4(1):5-13.

119. Black DM, Bilezikian JP, Ensrud KE, et al. One year of alendronate after one year of parathyroid hormone (1-84) for osteoporosis. *N Engl J Med*. 2005;353(6):555-565.

120. Nakamura T, Sugimoto T, Nakano T, et al. Randomized Teriparatide [human parathyroid hormone (PTH) 1-34] Once-Weekly Efficacy Research (TOWER) trial for examining the reduction in new vertebral fractures in subjects with primary osteoporosis and high fracture risk. *J Clin Endocrinol Metab*. 2012;97(9):3097-3106.

121. Neer RM, Arnaud CD, Zanchetta JR, et al. Effect of parathyroid hormone (1-34) on fractures and bone mineral density in postmenopausal women with osteoporosis. *N Engl J Med*. 2001; 344(19):1434-1441.

122. Tymlos (abaloparatide) [package insert]. Waltham, MA: Radius Health, Inc. 04/2017.

123. Miller PD, Hattersley G, Riis BJ, et al; ACTIVE Study Investigators. Effect of abaloparatide vs placebo on new vertebral fractures in postmenopausal women with osteoporosis: a randomized clinical trial. *JAMA*. 2016;316(7):722-733.

124. Cosman F, Miller PD, Williams GC, et al. Eighteen months of treatment with subcutaneous abaloparatide followed by 6 months of treatment with alendronate in postmenopausal women with osteoporosis: results of the ACTIVExtend Trial. *Mayo Clin Proc*. 2017;92(2):200-210.

125. Finkelstein JS, Hayes A, Hunzelman JL, et al. The effects of parathyroid hormone, alendronate, or both in men with osteoporosis. *N Engl J Med*. 2003;349(13):1216-1226.

126. Cosman F, Eriksen EF, Recknor C, et al. Effects of intravenous zoledronic acid plus subcutaneous teriparatide [rhPTH(1-34)]

in postmenopausal osteoporosis. *J Bone Miner Res*. 2011;26(3): 503-511.

127. Boonen S, Marin F, Obermayer-Pietsch B, et al. Effects of previous antiresorptive therapy on the bone mineral density response to two years of teriparatide treatment in postmenopausal women with osteoporosis. *J Clin Endocrinol Metab*. 2008;93(3):852-860.

128. Saag KG, Shane E, Boonen S, et al. Teriparatide or alendronate in glucocorticoid-induced osteoporosis. *N Engl J Med*. 2007; 357(20):2028-2039.

129. Saag KG, Zanchetta JR, Devogelaer JP, et al. Effects of teriparatide versus alendronate for treating glucocorticoid-induced osteoporosis: thirty-six-month results of a randomized, double-blind, controlled trial. *Arthritis Rheum*. 2009;60(11):3346-3355.

130. Dempster DW, Cosman F, Kurland ES, et al. Effects of daily treatment with parathyroid hormone on bone microarchitecture and turnover in patients with osteoporosis: a paired biopsy study. *J Bone Miner Res*. 2001;16(10):1846-1853.

9

10   Prevention and Treatment: Evolving Pathways and Therapeutic Targets

Over the past two decades, the master signals that integrate various endocrine, neuroendocrine, inflammatory, and mechanical stimuli, as well as several key molecules that coordinate activities of osteoblasts and osteoclasts during bone remodeling, have been identified.[1] This new understanding of the molecular and cellular factors has led to the identification of novel therapeutic targets and pathways, some of which are undergoing clinical trials.

The novel drugs currently under development can be categorized as either antiresorptive or anabolic agents. The former affect osteoclast physiology, while the latter affect osteoblast physiology. The potential therapeutic targets and mechanism of action of novel antiresorptive and anabolic agents are discussed below.

Osteoclast Physiology and Therapeutic Targets

Osteoclasts are large multinucleated cells derived from hematopoietic macrophage lineage.[2] Osteoclasts attach to bone surface to form a sealing zone with the help of $\alpha_v\beta_3$ integrin (**Figure 10.1**). Tyrosine src-kinase mediates multiple intracellular pathways regulating osteoclast activity, including the ability of osteoclasts to attach to bone to create a sealing zone on the bone surface, and to provide a highly enriched acidic microenvironment via proton pumps and chloride channels. A highly acidic environment is essential for catalytic activity of osteoclastic enzymes such as cathepsin K that degrade collagens and other bone matrix proteins. The differentiation of a fully activated osteoclast

FIGURE 10.1 — Osteoclast Physiology and Potential Therapeutic Targets

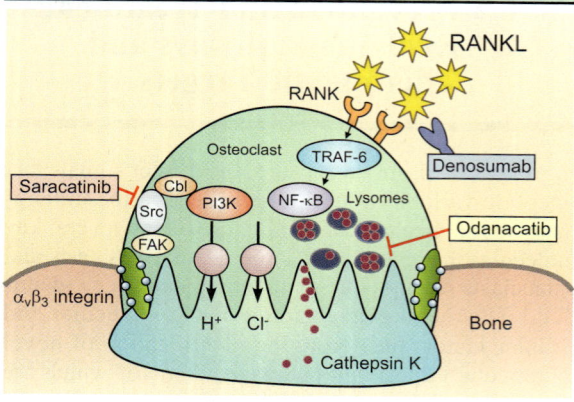

Key: FAK, focal adhesion kinase; NF-κB, nuclear factor kappa B; PI3K, phosphatidylinositol 3-kinase; RANK, receptor activator of NF-κB; RANKL, RANK ligand; TRAF-6, tumour necrosis factor receptor associated factor 6.

Adapted from Rachner TD, et al. *Lancet*. 2011;377(9773):1276-1287.

depends on the receptor activator of NF-κB ligand (RANKL) and the permissive role of macrophage-colony stimulating factor (M-CSF). Activation of the receptor RANK by RANKL results in the induction of several key regulatory transcription factors and enzymes. The result is resorption of bone. Blockade of this signaling pathway with denosumab, a humanized monoclonal antibody to RANKL, is one currently available therapeutic option for treating osteoporosis (see *Chapter 9*).

■ Therapeutic Targets

Novel antiresorptive agents have been developed that target critical osteoclast signaling and proteolytic pathways. These include:

- Cathepsin K
- Tyrosine src kinase.

Cathepsin K

The cysteine protease cathepsin K is a product of bone-resorbing osteoclasts, degrades collagen, and plays an essential role in the process of bone resorption.[3] Thus, cathepsin K inhibitors have emerged as novel therapeutic drugs. Agents with a high specificity and affinity for cathepsin K over other cathepsins (B, L, and S) that are widely expressed, particularly in the skin, are crucial for the development of this class of compounds. A clinical trial of balicatib, an inhibitor not entirely specific to cathepsin K, was discontinued due to a scleroderma-like skin condition that developed in study subjects. In a phase 2 trial of odanacatib, postmenopausal women with low BMD experienced a 5.5% increase in lumbar spine and a 3.2% increase in total hip BMD after receiving 2 years of 50 mg of oral odanacatib administered weekly.[4] BMD remained unchanged in the placebo group. At the 50-mg dose, odanacatib significantly reduced markers of bone resorption and formation. A phase 3 clinical trial involving more than 16,000 postmenopausal women with osteoporosis reported a significant reduction in both vertebral and nonvertebral fractures with odanacatib. However, the development of odanacatib was halted due to a significant increase in stroke events. It is unclear whether other cathepsin K inhibitors will be developed for the treatment of osteoporosis.

10

Tyrosine src kinase

Tyrosine src kinase mediates multiple intracellular pathways including the ability of osteoclasts to attach to bone to create a sealing zone on the bone surface and provide a highly enriched acidic microenvironment.[5] Therefore, a specific inhibitor of src kinase would be expected to have an antiresorptive effect. Saracatinib, a specific inhibitor of c-src kinase, is in the early stages of clinical development as an osteoporosis treatment.[6]

Osteoblast Physiology and Therapeutic Targets

At the molecular level, activation of the Wnt/β-catenin pathway is a master switch for osteoblastic differentiation (**Figure 10.2**).[7] LDL receptor-related proteins 5 and 6 (LRP5/6) act as co-receptors for a Wnt ligand to bind to the Frizzled receptor. Activation of this pathway results in degradation of GSK-3ß, stabilization of ß-catenin and its translocation to the nucleus, where it regulates transcription of osteoblastic genes. This key bone-anabolic pathway is negatively regulated by the Wnt inhibitors dickkopf-1 (DKK1) and sclerostin.[8,9] These Wnt inhibitors bind and block the Wnt co-receptors LRP5/6. DKK1 forms a complex with Kremen to bind LRP5/6, whereas sclerostin binds LRP5/6 directly.[10]

Manipulation of the calcium-sensing receptor (CaSR) represents another osteoblast anabolic strategy.[11] CaSR is located on parathyroid glands and controls PTH release to maintain serum calcium concentrations within a narrow physiologic range. Binding of PTH to its receptor enhances osteoblast function and bone formation (**Figure 10.2**).

■ Therapeutic Targets

Discoveries have led to a better understanding of osteoblast function and have uncovered potential therapeutic targets for osteoporosis. These targets include:
- Sclerostin
- DKK1
- The calcium-sending receptor (CaSR).

Sclerostin

Sclerostin is secreted by osteocytes and is an endogenous inhibitor of the Wnt/β-catenin anabolic pathway (**Figure 10.2**). The linking of inactivating mutations in the gene coding for sclerostin to two rare skeletal diseases with a high bone mass, van Buchem's disease and sclerosteosis, suggested a role for sclerostin

FIGURE 10.2 — Osteoblast Physiology and Potential Therapeutic Targets

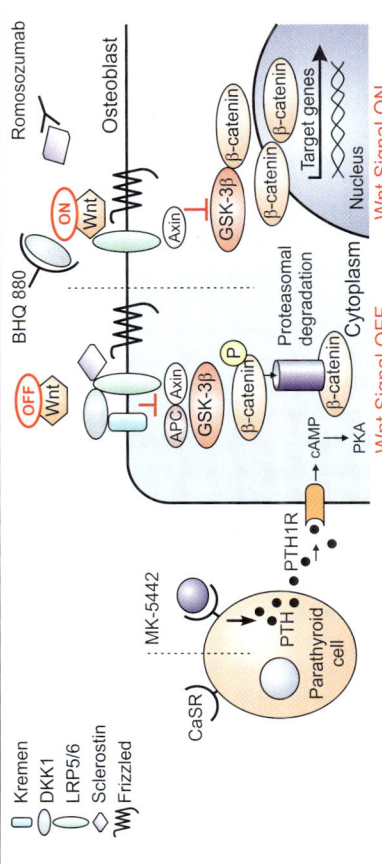

Key: APC, adenomatosis polyposis coli; cAMP, cyclic adenosine monophosphate; CaSR, calcium sensing receptor; DKK1, dickkopf-1; GSK, glycogen synthase kinase 3; LRP, low-density lipoprotein receptor-related protein; PKA, protein kinase A; PTH, parathyroid hormone; PTH1R, PTH 1 receptor.

Adapted from Rachner TD, et al. *Lancet*. 2011;377(9773):1276-1287.

in the homoeostasis of bone mass, and provided the rationale to target sclerostin with monoclonal antibodies to enhance bone formation. A therapeutic advantage of targeting sclerostin in the treatment of osteoporosis is that this protein is expressed solely by osteocytes. Therefore, a sclerostin-antagonizing drug would be expected to activate Wnt signaling in the adjacent osteoblasts and not other cell types, thereby likely producing a favorable side effect profile.

In a phase 2 clinical trial of postmenopausal women, compared with placebo, the anti-sclerostin antibody romosozumab significantly increased hip and spine BMD after 1 year of treatment.[12] Furthermore, romosozumab not only increased osteoblast activity as measured by bone turnover markers but also decreased bone resorption. A phase 3 trial enrolled over 7000 postmenopausal women with osteoporosis. Subjects were randomized to romosozumab vs placebo for 12 months followed by denosumab in all subjects for an additional 12 months. After the initial 12 months, subjects randomized to romosozumab had a 73% relative risk reduction in new vertebral fractures and a non-statistically significant 24% relative risk reduction in nonvertebral fractures.[13]

DKK1

DKK1 is another endogenous inhibitor of the Wnt/β-catenin anabolic pathway that regulates transcription of osteoblastic genes (**Figure 10.2**). Inhibition of DKK1 by neutralizing antibodies reduces bone loss in a model of rheumatoid arthritis and prevents the formation of osteolytic lesions and increases bone formation in a myeloma model.[14,15] The anti-DKK1 antibody, BHQ 880, is in the early stages of clinical development as a treatment for multiple myeloma. This medication may also increase BMD in osteoporosis patients but its effects in this population are unstudied.

The Calcium-Sensing Receptor (CaSR)

As noted previously, this receptor on parathyroid gland cells controls the release of PTH to maintain serum calcium concentrations within a narrow physiological range (**Figure 10.2**). Antagonism of the CaSR mimics hypocalcemia, evoking production of a short pulse of PTH and an increase in calcium levels. A high-amplitude PTH pulse followed by rapid normalization produces a bone-anabolic effect. Drugs that mimic hypocalcemia at the CaSR are described as calcilytic agents and represent a new class of bone-forming drugs.[16] A major practical obstacle in the development of these drugs has been their narrow therapeutic index. The development of several compounds has been discontinued due to sustained PTH secretion and effects suggestive of primary hyperparathyroidism. Newer calcilytic drugs with an improved pharmacological profile are currently being studied. A phase 2 trial testing the calcilytic drug MK-5442 in postmenopausal women with osteoporosis reported increase in markers of bone resorption.[17] However, no significant difference in spine BMD was found between the MK-5442 and placebo groups.

REFERENCES

1. Rachner TD, Khosla S, Hofbauer LC. Osteoporosis: now and the future. *Lancet*. 2011;377:1276-1287.

2. Henriksen K, Bollerslev J, Everts V, Karsdal MA. Osteoclast activity and subtypes as a function of physiology and pathology–implications for future treatments of osteoporosis. *Endocr Rev*. 2011;32:31-63.

3. Costa AG, Cusano NE, Silva BC, Cremers S, Bilezikian JP. Cathepsin K: its skeletal actions and role as a therapeutic target in osteoporosis. *Nat Rev Rheumatol*. 2011;7:447-456.

4. Bone H, McClung MR, Roux C, et al. Odanacatib, a cathepsin-K inhibitor for osteoporosis: a two-year study of postmenopausal women with low bone density. *J Bone Miner Res*. 2010; 25:937-947.

5. Miyazaki T, Sanjay A, Neff L, Tanaka S, Horne WC, Baron R. Src kinase activity is essential for osteoclast function. *J Biol Chem*. 2004;279:17660-17666.

6. Hannon RA, Clack G, Rimmer M, et al. Effects of the Src kinase inhibitor saracatinib (AZD0530) on bone turnover in healthy men: a randomized, double-blind, placebo-controlled,

10

multiple-ascending-dose phase I trial. *J Bone Miner Res*. 2010; 25:463-471.

7. Baron R, Rawadi G. Targeting the Wnt/beta-catenin pathway to regulate bone formation in the adult skeleton. *Endocrinology*. 2007;148:2635-2643.

8. Niida A, Hiroko T, Kasai M, et al. DKK1, a negative regulator of Wnt signaling, is a target of the beta-catenin/TCF pathway. *Oncogene*. 2004;23:8520-8526.

9. Li X, Zhang Y, Kang H, et al. Sclerostin binds to LRP5/6 and antagonizes canonical Wnt signaling. *J Biol Chem*. 2005;280: 19883-19887.

10. Mao B, Wu W, Davidson G, et al. Kremen proteins are Dickkopf receptors that regulate Wnt/beta-catenin signalling. *Nature*. 2002;417:664-667.

11. Brown EM, Gamba G, Riccardi D, et al. Cloning and characterization of an extracellular Ca(2+)-sensing receptor from bovine parathyroid. *Nature*. 1993;366:575-580.

12. McClung MR, Grauer A, Boonen S, et al. Inhibition of sclerostin with AMG 785 in postmenopausal women with low bone mineral density: phase II trial results. *J Bone Miner Res*. 2012;27(suppl 1). ASBMR Web site. http://www.asbmr.org/Meetings/AnnualMeeting/AbstractDetail.aspx?aid=9fa27a06-d9b5-4429-a95f-517048985173. Accessed May 26, 2017.

13. Cosman F, Crittenden DB, Adachi JD, et al. Romosozumab treatment in postmenopausal women with osteoporosis. *N Engl J Med*. 2016;375:1532-1543.

14. Diarra D, Stolina M, Polzer K, et al. Dickkopf-1 is a master regulator of joint remodeling. *Nat Med*. 2007;13:156-163.

15. Fulciniti M, Tassone P, Hideshima T, et al. Anti-DKK1 mAb (BHQ880) as a potential therapeutic agent for multiple myeloma. *Blood*. 2009;114:371-379.

16. Balan G, Bauman J, Bhattacharya S, et al. The discovery of novel calcium sensing receptor negative allosteric modulators. *Bioorg Med Chem Lett*. 2009;19:3328-3332.

17. Halse J, Greenspan SL, Cosman F, et al. A phase IIb, randomized, placebo-controlled, dose-ranging study of MK-5442 in the treatment of postmenopausal women with osteoporosis. *J Bone Miner Res*. 2012;27(suppl 1). ASBMR Web site. http://www.asbmr.org/Meetings/AnnualMeeting/AbstractDetail.aspx?aid=26e115c8-5d7f-4b37-b6f0-2cc6cb94fb0c. Accessed May 26, 2017.

11 Osteoporosis in Special Populations

Although osteoporosis has long been recognized as a disease affecting postmenopausal women, bone loss and increased fracture risk also occur in other patient populations. Secondary causes of bone loss should always be considered in patients who are diagnosed as having osteoporosis. In some studies, 20% to 30% of postmenopausal women and >50% of men with osteoporosis have a secondary cause, although the frequency of secondary osteoporosis is probably much lower in the general population. There are numerous causes of secondary bone loss, including adverse effects of drug therapy, endocrine disorders, renal disease, and cancer. In many cases, the adverse effects of osteoporosis are reversible with appropriate intervention. Therefore, in assessing the patient with presumed osteoporosis, it is important to consider other secondary causes and aggravating factors that may be reversible and amenable to therapy.

The reader is referred to the literature for more detailed information.

Osteoporosis in Men

Osteoporosis is becoming an increasingly important health problem in men. One in four men over the age of 60 years will suffer an osteoporotic fracture during their lifetime.[1] In men, as in women, increasing age and low BMD are the two most important independent risk factors for an initial vertebral or nonvertebral fracture. In addition, a systematic review of observational studies in men ≥50 years of age found that other consistent risk factors for low BMD and bone loss in men are smoking and low body weight or weight loss.[2]

Less common risk factors included physical/functional limitations and fracture after age 50. Furthermore, mortality after fracture is higher among men.[3] The progressive decrease in androgen and estrogen levels in elderly men appears to contribute to the age-related decrease in BMD.[4] Androgen deprivation therapy in men with prostate cancer is also an increasingly common cause associated with BMD loss and increased fracture risk (see below).[5]

While the diagnostic criteria for postmenopausal osteoporosis in women are well established, until recently, available data were not sufficient to suggest specific guidelines for the diagnosis and clinical management of the osteoporosis in elderly men. However, the Endocrine Society has released Clinical Guidelines on Osteoporosis in Men.[6] Because osteoporosis is less common in men, a thorough evaluation for secondary causes should be performed. These include hypogonadism, Cushing's syndrome, celiac disease, and primary hyperparathyroidism. Occult alcohol abuse is not uncommon as well. Approved pharmacologic agents for treatment of men at increased risk of fracture include alendronate, risedronate, zoledronic acid, teriparatide, and denosumab.

Low Bone Mass in Children

Although osteoporosis was once considered primarily a disease of the elderly, there is now increasing evidence that it has pediatric antecedents.[7] Although genetic factors play an important role in the attainment of an optimal adult (peak) bone mass and strength, lifestyle factors such as physical activity and nutrition are also important determinants of children's bone health.

Drug-related bone loss is also of concern in children and adolescents. For example, in one study, significant increases in markers of bone resorption were significantly increased in asthmatic children who were treated with inhaled glucocorticoids for at least 6 months compared with matched healthy controls.[8]

Long-term use of inhaled glucocorticoids in children also adversely affects BMD, especially in boys.[9] Low BMD and increased fractures have also been reported in children receiving chronic antiepileptic drug therapy.[10] Cancer and its treatment in children and teenagers adversely impact bone health.[11] Children with systemic illnesses that require systemic glucocorticoids, such as juvenile chronic arthritis, inflammatory bowel disease, and connective tissue disorders, such as systemic lupus erythematosus and myositis, experience a blunting of skeletal development in pre-adolescents, bone loss in developed skeletons, and a heightened risk of fractures.[12,13]

The diagnosis of osteoporosis in children should be made principally on fracture risk rather than BMD values measured by DXA.[14] Interpretation of BMD data must take into account the child's weight and pubertal status. Assuring sufficient calcium and adequate vitamin D is paramount for the developing skeleton and the need is heightened during adolescence. Children receiving glucocorticoids deserve special attention to dietary calcium, supplemental calcium and adequate vitamin D. In children 4 through 17 years of age receiving glucocorticoid treatment, the 2017 ACR guidelines for the prevention and treatment of glucocorticoid-induced osteoporosis recommend a calcium intake of 1000 mg/day and vitamin D intake of 600 IU/day. If a child has had an OP fracture and continues glucocorticoid treatment at a dose of ≥ 0.1 mg/kg/day for ≥ 3 months, treatment with a bisphosphonate is recommended. Oral contraceptives may provide a minimal bone boost in adolescent girls using chronic glucocorticoids. While bisphosphonates have been used successfully to treat children with osteogenesis imperfecta who experience fractures and have rarely been used in glucocorticoid associated bone disorders, they must be used cautiously in children due to their protracted skeletal effects and, particularly in girls of child-bearing potential, due to their mostly uncertain effects on a developing fetus.[15] Teriparatide is con-

11

traindicated in children because of the possible risk of osteosarcoma in individuals with open epiphyses. Abaloparatide is not recommended in patients at increased risk of osteosarcoma, including those with open epiphyses.

Osteoporosis in Diabetics

Although the pathologic processes that may lead to abnormal bone metabolism and increased fracture risk in diabetic patients is not yet fully understood, accumulating evidence indicates that type 1 and type 2 diabetes are associated with increased risk of fracture.[16,17] The accumulation of advanced glycation end products (AGEs) of collagen fibrils and defects in bone mineralization have been proposed to contribute to increased fracture risk. Patients with recent onset of type 1 diabetes mellitus may have impaired bone formation because of the absence of the anabolic effects of insulin and amylin, whereas in long-standing type 1 diabetes mellitus, vascular complications may account for low bone mass and increased fracture risk. Patients with type 2 diabetes mellitus display an increased fracture risk despite a higher BMD.[18] The use of thiazolidinediones is associated with increased risk of fracture.[19]

Although routine screening or initiation of preventive medications for osteoporosis in patients with type 1 or type 2 diabetes is not recommended at the present time, recommendations should be given regarding adequate dietary calcium intake, regular exercise, and avoidance of other potential risk factors such as smoking in addition to optimal glycemic control. In patients who have risk factors for osteoporosis, or in those who present with fractures, evaluation of bone density should be performed and appropriate preventive or therapeutic interventions should be prescribed.

Renal Bone Disease

Mechanisms of bone loss in patients with chronic kidney disease (CKD) are complex. Secondary hyperparathyroidism, tertiary hyperparathyroidism, hyperphosphatemia, vitamin D deficiency, and chronic metabolic acidosis all have profound effects on bone homeostasis.[20] Both osteomalacia and adynamic bone disease can complicate diagnosis. Before aluminum was recognized as having adverse effects on bone, aluminum-containing phosphate binders and aluminum contaminated dialysate water also contributed to significant bone disease. The term chronic kidney disease-mineral and bone disorder (CKD-MBD) has been proposed to encompass the different types of bone disease commonly seen in patients with CKD.[21]

Bone turnover rate is often used as a surrogate for bone health in CKD patients (**Figure 11.1**). Tools to assess bone turnover include bone biopsy, an accurate but cumbersome and painful procedure that determines rates of bone formation, bone resorption and mineralization. As more specific and sensitive intact PTH (iPTH) assays have been developed, bone biopsy is now rarely performed, although CKD remains one of the few residual indications for this procedure. While iPTH assays are universally available, this test only provides a rough estimate of bone turnover.

Normal reference ranges of iPTH (10-65 pg/mL) do not apply to patients with advanced CKD due to a syndrome of PTH resistance. CKD patients with normal bone turnover, as measured by bone biopsy, have iPTH levels that range between normal to 500 pg/mL depending on the degree of renal dysfunction.[22,23] Lower iPTH is associated with the low-turnover states of adynamic bone disease and osteomalacia, and places these patients at highest fracture risk.[24] Excessive $1,25(OH)_2D_3$ replacement is a common cause.[25] Intact PTH levels greater than 500 pg/mL are associated with high bone turnover, osteitis cystica, and increased fracture risk. The KDOQI guidelines

11

FIGURE 11.1 — PTH and Bone Turnover in CKD

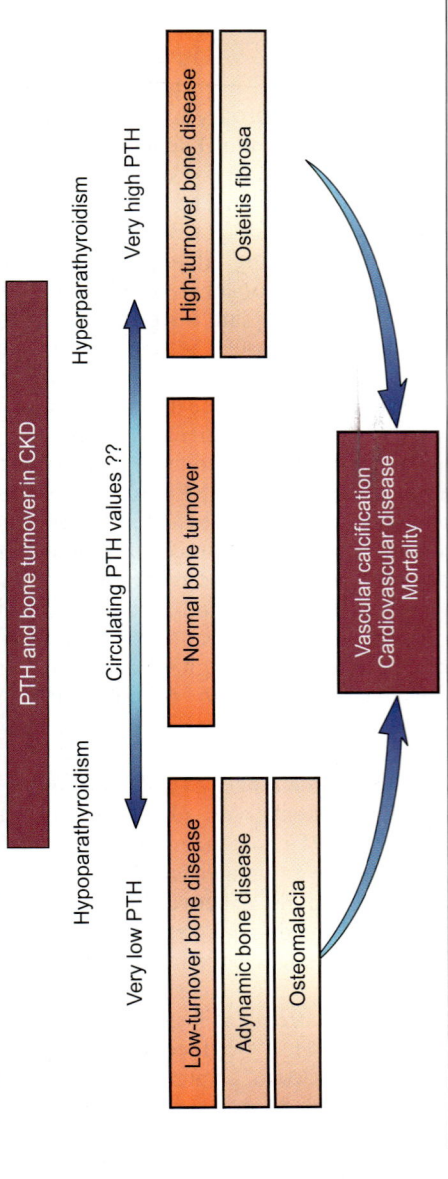

Drüeke TB. *Kidney Int.* 2008;73:674-676.

recommend a PTH concentration between 150 to 300 pg/mL for dialysis patients.[26] Adequate $1,25(OH)_2D_3$ replacement and phosphate binders will often lower iPTH levels. Persistent iPTH greater than 800 pg/mL despite aggressive measures to lower bone turnover is a sign of tertiary hyperparathyroidism, a condition of parathyroid gland hyperplasia and autonomous iPTH secretion. Four-gland parathyroidectomy followed by one-half parathyroid gland autotransplantation into the sternocleidomastoid muscle or forearm is the preferred treatment in patients with tertiary hyperparathyroidism in the setting of severe bone disease.[23]

Treatment of bone disease in CKD patients is challenging. Cinacalcet, a calcimimetic that modulates the calcium sensing receptor signaling, lowers iPTH in patients with high bone turnover.[27] Bisphosphonates are not well studied in this population and their use is generally discouraged. A potential risk of bisphosphonates is renal toxicity, especially in patients with minimal renal reserve but not yet requiring dialysis. Denosumab has been studied in patients with mild CKD, but its benefits in patients with more severe CKD (GFR <30 mL/min) or in patients on dialysis are unknown.[28] There is anecdotal data suggesting a putative role for teriparatide in adynamic bone disease.[29]

Drugs That Increase the Risk of Fracture

11

■ **Proton Pump Inhibitors**
Gastric proton pump inhibitors (PPIs) are widely used in the treatment of dyspepsia. According to several studies, use of PPIs, particularly at high dose, was associated with increased risk of fracture.[30,31] Although the mechanisms for this effect are not fully understood, PPIs may interfere with calcium absorption through induction of hypochlorhydria. This would be consistent with the finding in some but not all studies that H_2 inhibitors and other antacids were also associated with increased fracture risk.

■ **Selective Serotonin Inhibitors**

Depression and osteoporotic fractures are common conditions among elderly persons. Selective serotonin reuptake inhibitors (SSRIs) are frequently used in the treatment of depression in this population. SSRIs have been associated with lower BMD and increased risk of fracture in older individuals.[32] Active serotoninergic pathways have been discovered in osteoblasts that reduce osteoblast activity.[33] This has raised concern about the use of SSRIs in patients who are at higher fracture risk and the need for more careful bone surveillance in this population.

■ **Glucocorticoids**

The adverse effects of glucocorticoids on bone fragility and fracture risk has been known for many years. Glucocorticoids affect bones adversely both through an increase in bone resorption and perhaps most importantly due to osteocyte and osteoblast apoptosis leading to reduced bone formation (**Figure 11.2**).[34,35] Glucocorticoid-induced osteoporosis (GIOP), which is estimated to affect approximately 50% of patients treated for 6 months or longer, is probably the most common form of secondary osteoporosis.[36] Glucocorticoids initially affect primarily trabecular bone at sites such as the spine and trochanter. Bone loss is accelerated during early use and has been reported to be as high a 20% reduction in BMD in the first 6 to 12 months, depending on the glucocorticoid dose, although a 3% to 5% decline in trabecular BMD is more common.[37] The estimated cumulative fracture incidence, predominantly at the spine and ribs, is approximately 35%, while the risk of hip fracture in glucocorticoid users is almost double that in non-users. Daily oral doses as low as 2.5 mg to 7.5 mg (prednisone equivalents) can increase fracture risk.[38] Even inhaled glucocorticoids and intra-articular preparations have been associated with a reduction in biochemical measures of bone formation, suggestion the absence of a truly safe dose.[39]

FIGURE 11.2 — The Pathophysiology of GIOP

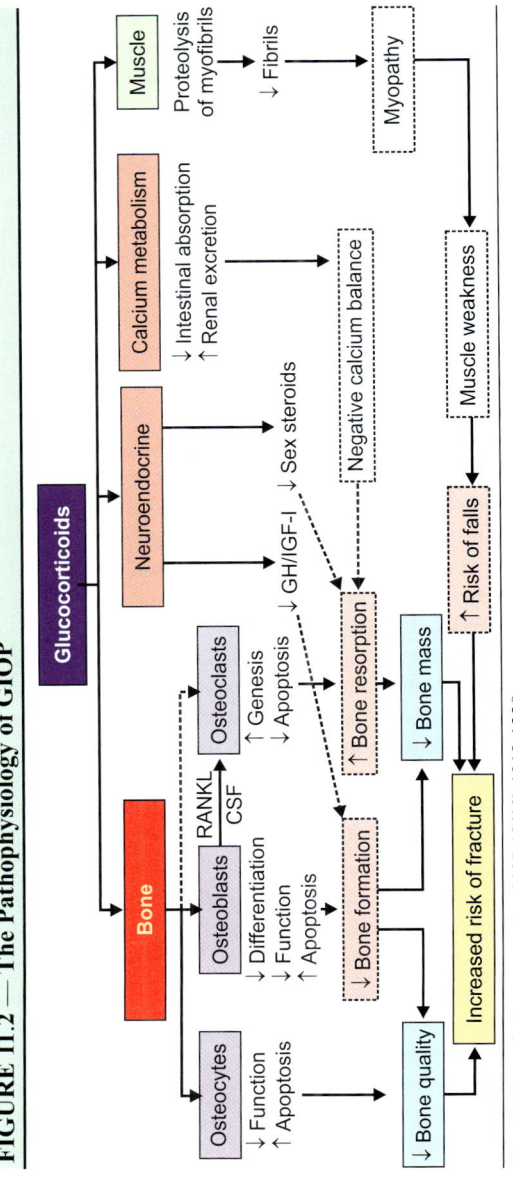

Canalis E, et al. *Osteoporos Int.* 2007;18(10):1319-1328.

11

The effects of the underlying glucocorticoid requiring illnesses, such as one of the most common disorders utilizing glucocorticoids, rheumatoid arthritis, can also have direct deleterious effects on bone.[38,40] However, it is not only the dose but also the duration of treatment that can result in GIOP. The risk of fracture appears to be at a maximum within 6 months of starting treatment and then generally decreases after therapy is stopped. Glucocorticoid users fracture at a higher (better) BMD than non-users, likely due to the direct toxic effect of glucocorticoids on osteoblasts and osteocytes.[41] Approved interventions for the prevention and treatment of GIOP include alendronate, etidronate (not in the United States), risedronate, zoledronic acid, and teriparatide (see *Chapter 9*).

The ACR first published recommendations for the prevention and treatment of GIOP in 1996, with subsequent updates released in 2001, 2010, and 2017. These guidelines address initial assessment and reassessment of clinical fracture risk in patients beginning or continuing long-term glucocorticoid treatment, as well as the benefits and risks of lifestyle modifications and pharmacologic treatment. The 2017 ACR guidelines recommend that in all adults and children, an initial clinical fracture risk assessment be performed at least within 6 months of the initiation of long-term glucocorticoid treatment.[42] Assessment should include a history with details of glucocorticoid use, an evaluation for falls, fractures, fragility, other risk factors for fracture, and other clinical comorbidities, a physical examination, testing of muscle strength, and an assessment for other clinical findings of undiagnosed fracture. Additional testing is recommended based on age (**Figure 11.3**), and may include BMD testing and risk assessment of major osteoporotic fracture calculated by FRAX. In all adults and children who continue glucocorticoid treatment, a clinical fracture risk reassessment should be performed every 12 months (**Figure 11.4**).

Recommendations for all patients receiving glucocorticoid treatment include optimizing calcium

FIGURE 11.3 — ACR Guidelines: Initial Fracture Risk Assessment

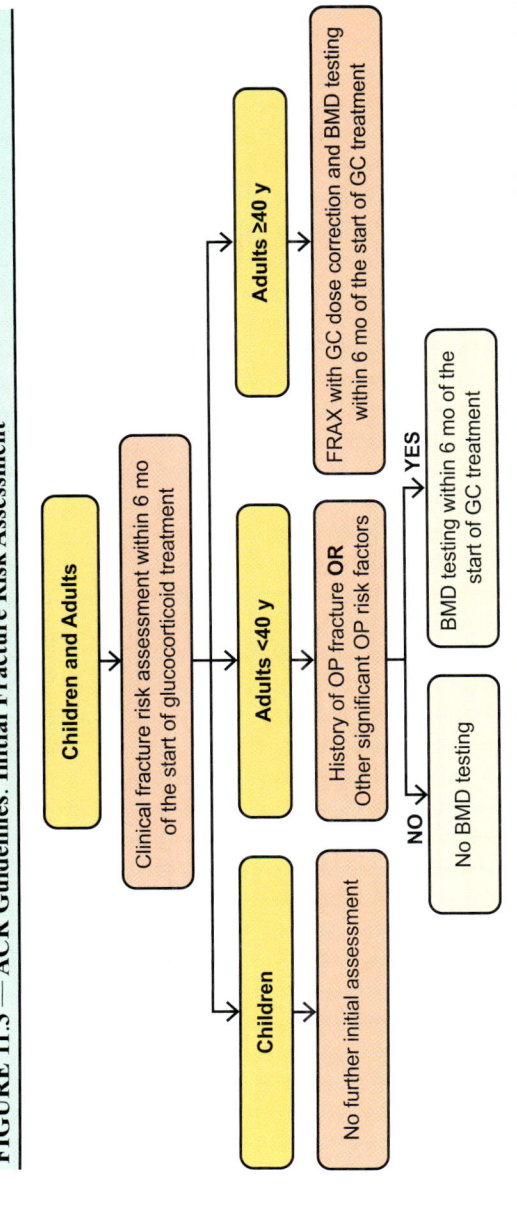

Buckley L, et al. *Arthritis Rheumatol.* 2017. Epub ahead of print.

FIGURE 11.4 — ACR Guidelines: Reassessment of Fracture Risk

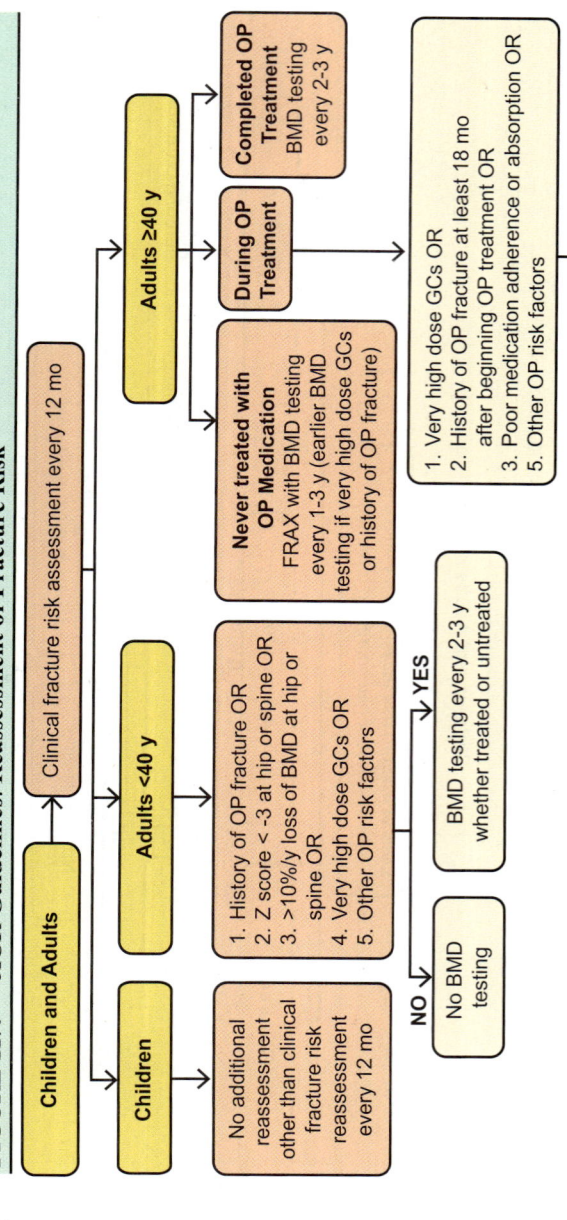

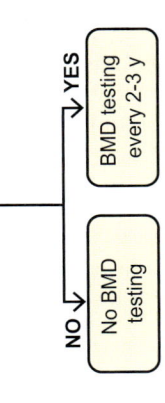

NO → No BMD testing

YES → BMD testing every 2-3 y

Buckley L, et al. *Arthritis Rheumatol.* 2017. Epub ahead of print.

11

intake (1000-1200 mg/day) and vitamin D intake (600-800 IU/day; serum level ≥20 ng/mL), in addition to lifestyle modifications, which include a balanced diet, maintaining weight in the recommended range, regular weight-bearing or resistance training exercise, smoking cessation, and limited alcohol intake. Initial pharmacologic treatment recommendations for adults are shown in **Figure 11.5**. Women ≥40 years of age and not of childbearing potential and men ≥40 years of age who are at moderate-to-high risk of fracture should be treated with an oral bisphosphonate in addition to calcium and vitamin D intake. Other suggested therapies, in order of preference, include IV bisphosphonates, teriparatide, denosumab, and raloxifene for postmenopausal women if no other therapy is available. For adults <40 years of age at moderate-to-high risk of fracture, an oral bisphosphonate should be used rather than the patient receiving no additional treatment beyond calcium and vitamin D. For patients in whom oral bisphosphonates are not appropriate, the same alternative medications listed for adults ≥40 years of age are recommended, except for raloxifene. Please refer to the 2017 ACR guidelines for follow-up recommendations and additional treatment recommendations in special populations.

■ Thiazolidinediones

Rosiglitazone and pioglitazone are peroxisome proliferator-activated receptor γ (PPARγ) agonists that increase peripheral insulin sensitivity and are approved for treatment of type 2 diabetes. PPARγ activation also steers mesenchymal stem cells toward an adipocyte and away from an osteoblast fate. As a consequence, PPARγ agonists have been associated with bone loss and fractures.[19] Because of reported adverse cardiovascular side effects, especially with rosiglitazone, and the weight-retaining effects of this class of medication, the use of PPARγ agonists has declined.

■ Transplant Anti-rejection Medications

Improved survival rates in organ or cell transplant recipients have been accompanied by increased recognition of adverse skeletal effects including fractures.[43] Pre-transplantation bone disease and immunosuppressive therapy, such as glucocorticoids and calcineurin inhibitors, result in rapid bone loss and increased fracture rates early after transplantation. Transplant patients deserve careful surveillance of bone mass. Small clinical trials and observational studies support the use of conventional osteoporosis treatments, specifically bisphosphonates, in this population.

■ Cancer Chemotherapy

Cytotoxic drugs can have wide ranging effects on bone. Most of the time, the effects on bone occur through indirect mechanisms such as gonadal toxicity resulting in lower sex steroids. In particular, aromatase inhibitors and androgen deprivation therapy (see below) reduce sex steroids and decrease BMD (**Figure 11.6**). Glucocorticoids are also a part of the chemotherapy armamentarium that have profound negative effects on bone. However, cytotoxic drugs such as methotrexate (although not in the doses used to manage inflammatory disorders) and imatinib have been shown to have direct effects on bone and reduce BMD.[44,45]

■ Aromatase Inhibitors

Aromatase inhibitors (AIs) have become standard therapy in women with breast cancer with estrogen-responsive disease. Medications in this class, letrozole, anastrozole, and exemestane, block the conversion of androstenedione to estrone, and testosterone to estradiol. As expected, AIs increase bone turnover and bone loss in women who are already at risk for fracture. The Arimidex, Tamoxifen, Alone or in Combination (ATAC) trial showed that fracture rates were significantly higher in women assigned to anastrozole (Arimidex) (11.0%) vs the selective estrogen receptor modulator (SERM) tamoxifen (7.7%) after 5 years of therapy.[46] Other clinical trials evaluating AIs vs tamoxifen have reported similar findings.[47-49]

Prevention of bone loss and fracture is critical in women treated with AIs. Ensuring adequate dietary cal-

11

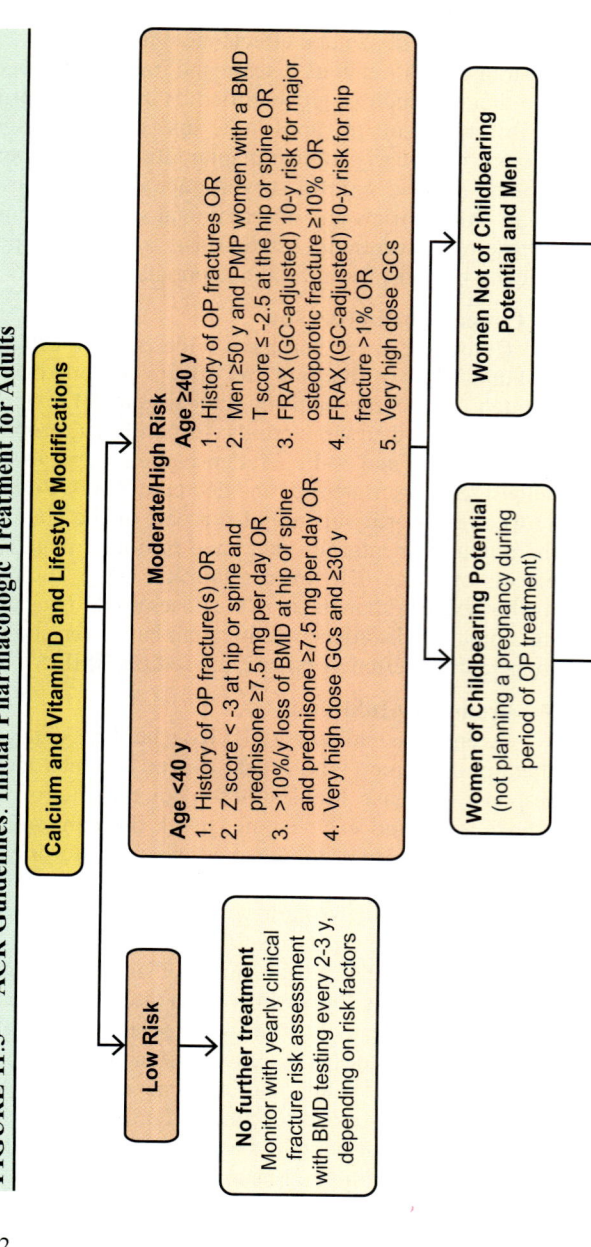

FIGURE 11.5 — ACR Guidelines: Initial Pharmacologic Treatment for Adults

Calcium and Vitamin D and Lifestyle Modifications

Low Risk

No further treatment
Monitor with yearly clinical fracture risk assessment with BMD testing every 2-3 y, depending on risk factors

Moderate/High Risk

Age <40 y
1. History of OP fracture(s) OR
2. Z score < -3 at hip or spine and prednisone ≥7.5 mg per day OR
3. >10%/y loss of BMD at hip or spine and prednisone ≥7.5 mg per day OR
4. Very high dose GCs and ≥30 y

Age ≥40 y
1. History of OP fractures OR
2. Men ≥50 y and PMP women with a BMD T score ≤ -2.5 at the hip or spine OR
3. FRAX (GC-adjusted) 10-y risk for major osteoporotic fracture ≥10% OR
4. FRAX (GC-adjusted) 10-y risk for hip fracture >1% OR
5. Very high dose GCs

Women of Childbearing Potential
(not planning a pregnancy during period of OP treatment)

Women Not of Childbearing Potential and Men

Treat with an oral bisphosphonate
Second-line therapy: **teriparatide**
Other suggested therapies (in order of preference) for high-risk women for whom the previous drugs are not appropriate:
IV bisphosphonates
denosumab

Treat with an oral bisphosphonate
Other suggested therapies (in order of preference):
IV bisphosphonates
teriparatide
denosumab
raloxifene for PMP women if no other therapy is available

Buckley L, et al. *Arthritis Rheumatol*. 2017. Epub ahead of print.

11

283

FIGURE 11.6 — BMD Loss With Cancer Therapies

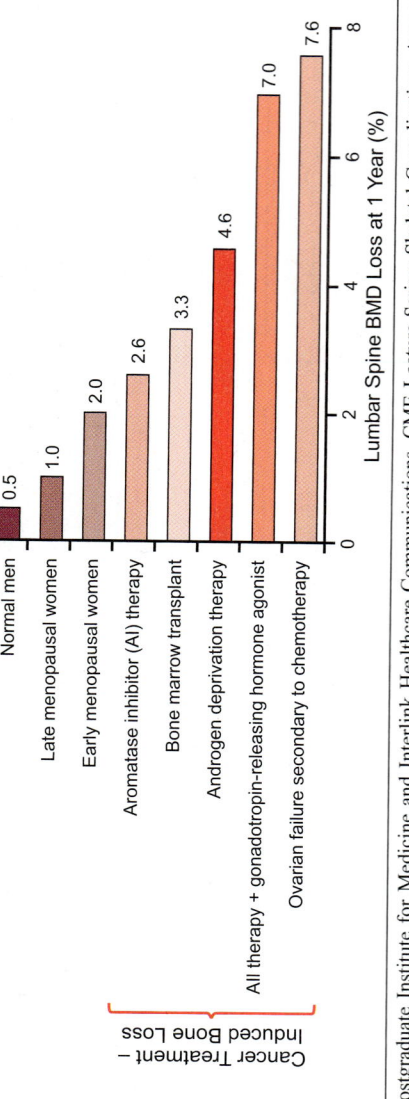

Postgraduate Institute for Medicine and Interlink Healthcare Communications. CME Lecture Series: Skeletal Complications Across the Cancer Continuum. Slide/Lecture Kit release date: June 2005.

cium intake and vitamin D is important. The addition of oral bisphosphonates (risedronate and ibandronate) have been reported to protect against BMD loss in women receiving AIs.[50-52] Trials evaluated zoledronic acid, 4 mg IV every 6 months vs delayed zoledronic acid only when the spine or hip T-score crossed the -2.0 threshold or when a fracture occurred. After 61 months, the upfront treatment group-adjusted mean BMD was 8.9% greater in the lumbar spine and 6.7% great in the hip compared with the delayed-treatment group.[53] Denosumab is another option to prevent bone loss with AIs. At the standard osteoporosis treatment dose of 60 mg subcutaneously every 6 months, BMD was 7.6% greater in the treatment group compared with the placebo group after 24 months.[54] No studies have been sufficiently powered to demonstrate fracture reduction or have compared the efficacy of antiresorptive medications in this clinical setting.

■ Androgen Deprivation Therapy

Androgen deprivation therapy (ADT) is part of standard therapy in men with castrate-sensitive prostate cancer. Gonadotropin-releasing hormone (GnRH) agonists and androgen receptor antagonists are commonly used. As expected, ADT significantly reduces bone mass and increases fracture risk in men with prostate cancer. The relative risk for experiencing any clinical fracture was reported to be 1.21 (95% CI, 1.14-1.29; $P<0.001$) in men with early disease stage disease receiving a GnRH agonist.[5]

As with women receiving AIs, men who receive ADT require adequate dietary calcium and vitamin D. Zoledronic acid at a dose of 4 mg IV every 3 months for 1 year increased BMD 5.6% compared with a 2.2% decrease in patients assigned placebo.[55] Denosumab has also been reported to protect against bone loss. Bone density increased 5.6% in the denosumab group (60 mg subcutaneously every 6 months) while BMD decreased 1.0% in the placebo group after 24 months of treatment.[56] The SERM toremifene not only increased BMD in men receiving ADT but also significantly

11

reduced the incidence of fracture.[57] Toremifene is neither EMA nor FDA approved for preventing BMD loss in men receiving ADT.

■ Anti-epileptic Drugs

Many anti-epileptic drugs (AEDs) have been associated with reduced BMD and an increased fracture risk.[58,59] Increased falls with seizures themselves may confound the association AEDs with fracture risk. However, convincing evidence supports AEDs' direct effects on bone homeostasis. One example is the alteration in vitamin D metabolism. Phenytoin, carbamazepine, and phenobarbital increase the activity of several cytochrome P450 enzymes involved in the metabolism and inactivation of vitamin D.[60,61] A consequence is impaired calcium absorption and secondary hyperparathyroidism. Phenytoin and carbamazepine have been reported to decrease osteoblast proliferation.[62] Valproate may inhibit longitudinal bone growth in children by inhibiting cartilage formation.[63] Many of the newer AEDs may in fact have a lower risk for fracture but more study is needed.[64]

Select AEDs place patients at higher fracture risk and should therefore undergo more frequent screening for vitamin D deficiency and low bone mass. Furthermore, these patients should receive adequate dietary calcium and vitamin D. Patients discovered to have low bone mass, osteoporosis or have a high fracture risk should be offered therapy.

■ Heparin

Studies have shown that long-term use of heparin for thromboembolism prevention, especially during pregnancy, is associated with low BMD.[65,66] Increasing use of long-term heparin for management of antiphospholipid antibody syndrome during pregnancy has heightened concern of this risk. Mechanisms of heparin-induced bone loss are unknown.

■ Sodium Glucose Co-transporter-2 Inhibitors

Sodium glucose co-transporter-2 (SGLT2) inhibitors operate by decreasing renal reabsorption of filtered glucose in the proximal tubule, resulting in glycosuria and lower blood sugars. A recent concern of these diabetes medications is an increased fracture risk. Post-hoc analyses of the CANVAS trial reported that 4.0% of subjects randomized to the SGLT2 inhibitor cana-gliflozin experienced fractures compared with 2.6% in the control subjects (HR 1.51 [95% CI, 1.04-2.19]).[67] A reduction in bone mass and orthostatic hypotension leading to more falls has been proposed as contributors to excess fractures. The effects of other SGLT2 inhibitors empagliflozin and dapagliflozin on bone health and fractures have not been rigorously studied. Avoidance of SGLT2 inhibitors in patients with high fracture risk is a reasonable approach at this time.

REFERENCES

1. Nguyen TV, Eisman JA, Kelly PJ, Sambrook PN. Risk factors for osteoporotic fractures in elderly men. *Am J Epidemiol.* 1996;144:255-263.

2. Papaioannou A, Kennedy CC, Cranney A, et al. Risk factors for low BMD in healthy men age 50 years or older: a systematic review. *Osteoporos Int.* 2009;20:507-518.

3. Kanis JA, Oden A, Johnell O, De Laet C, Jonsson B, Oglesby AK. The components of excess mortality after hip fracture. *Bone.* 2003;32:468-473.

4. Falahati-Nini A, Riggs BL, Atkinson EJ, O'Fallon WM, Eastell R, Khosla S. Relative contributions of testosterone and estrogen in regulating bone resorption and formation in normal elderly men. *J Clin Invest.* 2000;106:1553-1560.

5. Smith MR, Lee WC, Brandman J, Wang Q, Botteman M, Pashos CL. Gonadotropin-releasing hormone agonists and fracture risk: a claims-based cohort study of men with non-metastatic prostate cancer. *J Clin Oncol.* 2005;23:7897-7903.

6. Watts NB, Adler RA, Bilezikian, et al. Osteoporosis in men: An Endocrine Society Clinical Practice Guideline. *J Clin Endocrinol Metab.* 2012;97(6):1802-1822.

7. Bianchi ML. Osteoporosis in children and adolescents. *Bone.* 2007;41:486-495.

8. Sorva R, Turpeinen M, Juntunen-Backman K, Karonen SL, Sorva A. Effects of inhaled budesonide on serum markers of bone metabolism in children with asthma. *J Allergy Clin Immunol.* 1992;90:808-815.

11

9. Kelly HW, Van Natta ML, Covar RA, Tonascia J, Green RP, Strunk RC. Effect of long-term corticosteroid use on bone mineral density in children: a prospective longitudinal assessment in the childhood Asthma Management Program (CAMP) study. *Pediatrics*. 2008;122:e53-e61.

10. Coppola G, Fortunato D, Auricchio G, et al. Bone mineral density in children, adolescents, and young adults with epilepsy. *Epilepsia*. 2009;50:2140-2146.

11. Wasilewski-Masker K, Kaste SC, Hudson MM, Esiashvili N, Mattano LA, Meacham LR. Bone mineral density deficits in survivors of childhood cancer: long-term follow-up guidelines and review of the literature. *Pediatrics*. 2008;121:e705-e713.

12. Leonard MB. Glucocorticoid-induced osteoporosis in children: impact of the underlying disease. *Pediatrics*. 2007;119(suppl 2):S166-S174.

13. Huber AM, Gaboury I, Cabral DA, et al. Prevalent vertebral fractures among children initiating glucocorticoid therapy for the treatment of rheumatic disorders. *Arthritis Care Res (Hoboken)*. 2010;62:516-526.

14. Skeletal Health Assessment In Children from Infancy to Adolescence. 2013 ISCD Official Position. The International Society for Clinical Densitometry Web Site. Last modified September 2, 2014. https://www.iscd.org/official-positions/2013-iscd-official-positions-pediatric/. Accessed May 26, 2017.

15. Bachrach LK, Ward LM. Clinical review: Bisphosphonate use in childhood osteoporosis. *J Clin Endocrinol Metab*. 2009;94: 400-409.

16. Vestergaard P. Discrepancies in bone mineral density and fracture risk in patients with type 1 and type 2 diabetes–a meta-analysis. *Osteoporos Int*. 2007;18:427-444.

17. Bonds DE, Larson JC, Schwartz AV, et al. Risk of fracture in women with type 2 diabetes: the Women's Health Initiative Observational Study. *J Clin Endocrinol Metab*. 2006;91:3404-3410.

18. van Daele PL, Stolk RP, Burger H, et al. Bone density in non-insulin-dependent diabetes mellitus. The Rotterdam Study. *Ann Intern Med*. 1995;122:409-414.

19. Habib ZA, Havstad SL, Wells K, Divine G, Pladevall M, Williams LK. Thiazolidinedione use and the longitudinal risk of fractures in patients with type 2 diabetes mellitus. *J Clin Endocrinol Metab*. 2010;95:592-600.

20. Moe S, Drueke T, Cunningham J, et al. Definition, evaluation, and classification of renal osteodystrophy: a position statement from Kidney Disease: Improving Global Outcomes (KDIGO). *Kidney Int.* 2006;69:1945-1953.

21. Miller PD. Bone disease in CKD: a focus on osteoporosis diagnosis and management. *Am J Kidney Dis.* 2014;64(2):290-304.

22. Quarles LD, Lobaugh B, Murphy G. Intact parathyroid hormone overestimates the presence and severity of parathyroid-mediated osseous abnormalities in uremia. *J Clin Endocrinol Metab.* 1992;75:145-150.

23. Eknoyan G, Levin A, Levin NW. K/DOQI clinical practice guidelines for bone metabolism and disease in chronic kidney disease. *Am J Kidney Dis.* 2003;42:S1-S201.

24. Coco M, Rush H. Increased incidence of hip fractures in dialysis patients with low serum parathyroid hormone. *Am J Kidney Dis.* 2000;36:1115-1121.

25. Malluche HH, Monier-Faugere MC. Risk of adynamic bone disease in dialyzed patients. *Kidney Int Suppl.* 1992;38:S62-S67.

26. National Kidney Foundation. KDOQI clinical practice guidelines for bone metabolism and disease in chronic kidney disease. *Am J Kidney Dis.* 2003;42(4 suppl 3):S1/S201.

27. Moe SM, Chertow GM, Coburn JW, et al. Achieving NKF-K/DOQI bone metabolism and disease treatment goals with cinacalcet HCl. *Kidney Int.* 2005;67:760-771.

28. Jamal SA, Ljunggren O, Stehman-Breen C, et al. Effects of denosumab on fracture and bone mineral density by level of kidney function. *J Bone Miner Res.* 2011;26:1829-1835.

29. Cejka D, Kodras K, Bader T, Haas M. Treatment of Hemodialysis-Associated Adynamic Bone Disease with Teriparatide (PTH(1-34)): A Pilot Study. *Kidney Blood Press Res.* 2010;33(3):221-226.

30. Vestergaard P, Rejnmark L, Mosekilde L. Proton pump inhibitors, histamine H_2 receptor antagonists, and other antacid medications and the risk of fracture. *Calcif Tissue Int.* 2006;79:76-83.

31. Yang YX, Lewis JD, Epstein S, Metz DC. Long-term proton pump inhibitor therapy and risk of hip fracture. *JAMA.* 2006; 296:2947-2953.

32. Wu Q, Bencaz AF, Hentz JG, Crowell MD. Selective serotonin reuptake inhibitor treatment and risk of fractures: a meta-analysis of cohort and case-control studies. *Osteoporos Int.* 2012;23:365-375.

11

33. Warden SJ, Robling AG, Sanders MS, Bliziotes MM, Turner CH. Inhibition of the serotonin (5-hydroxytryptamine) transporter reduces bone accrual during growth. *Endocrinology*. 2005;146:685-693.

34. Canalis E, Bilezikian JP, Angeli A, Giustina A. Perspectives on glucocorticoid-induced osteoporosis. *Bone*. 2004;34:593-598.

35. Manolagas SC, Weinstein RS. New developments in the pathogenesis and treatment of steroid-induced osteoporosis. *J Bone Miner Res*. 1999;14:1061-1066.

36. Canalis E, Mazziotti G, Giustina A, Bilezikian JP. Glucocorticoid-induced osteoporosis: pathophysiology and therapy. *Osteoporos Int*. 2007;18:1319-1328.

37. Bijlsma JW, Saag KG, Buttgereit F, da Silva JA. Developments in glucocorticoid therapy. *Rheum Dis Clin North Am*. 2005;31:1-17, vii.

38. van Staa TP, Leufkens HG, Abenhaim L, Zhang B, Cooper C. Oral corticosteroids and fracture risk: relationship to daily and cumulative doses. *Rheumatology (Oxford)*. 2000;39:1383-1389.

39. Emkey RD, Lindsay R, Lyssy J, Weisberg JS, Dempster DW, Shen V. The systemic effect of intraarticular administration of corticosteroid on markers of bone formation and bone resorption in patients with rheumatoid arthritis. *Arthritis Rheum*. 1996;39:277-282.

40. Cooper C, Coupland C, Mitchell M. Rheumatoid arthritis, corticosteroid therapy and hip fracture. *Ann Rheum Dis*. 1995;54:49-52.

41. Van Staa TP, Laan RF, Barton IP, Cohen S, Reid DM, Cooper C. Bone density threshold and other predictors of vertebral fracture in patients receiving oral glucocorticoid therapy. *Arthritis Rheum*. 2003;48:3224-3229.

42. Buckley L, Guyatt G, Fink HA, et al. 2017 American College of Rheumatology guideline for the prevention and treatment of glucocorticoid-induced osteoporosis [published online ahead of print June 6, 2017]. *Arthritis Rheumatol*. doi: 10.1002/art.40137.

43. Cohen A, Shane E. Osteoporosis after solid organ and bone marrow transplantation. *Osteoporos Int*. 2003;14:617-630.

44. Schwartz AM, Leonidas JC. Methotrexate osteopathy. *Skeletal Radiol*. 1984;11:13-16.

45. Berman E, Nicolaides M, Maki RG, et al. Altered bone and mineral metabolism in patients receiving imatinib mesylate. *N Engl J Med*. 2006;354:2006-2013.

46. Howell A, Cuzick J, Baum M, et al. Results of the ATAC (Arimidex, Tamoxifen, Alone or in Combination) trial after completion of 5 years' adjuvant treatment for breast cancer. *Lancet.* 2005;365:60-62.

47. Rabaglio M, Sun Z, Price KN, et al. Bone fractures among postmenopausal patients with endocrine-responsive early breast cancer treated with 5 years of letrozole or tamoxifen in the BIG 1-98 trial. *Ann Oncol.* 2009;20:1489-1498.

48. Coleman RE, Banks LM, Girgis SI, et al. Skeletal effects of exemestane on bone-mineral density, bone biomarkers, and fracture incidence in postmenopausal women with early breast cancer participating in the Intergroup Exemestane Study (IES): a randomised controlled study. *Lancet Oncol.* 2007;8:119-127.

49. Jakesz R, Jonat W, Gnant M, et al. Switching of postmenopausal women with endocrine-responsive early breast cancer to anastrozole after 2 years' adjuvant tamoxifen: combined results of ABCSG trial 8 and ARNO 95 trial. *Lancet.* 2005;366:455-462.

50. Greenspan SL, Brufsky A, Lembersky BC, et al. Risedronate prevents bone loss in breast cancer survivors: a 2-year, randomized, double-blind, placebo-controlled clinical trial. *J Clin Oncol.* 2008;26:2644-2652.

51. Lester JE, Dodwell D, Purohit OP, et al. Prevention of anastrozole-induced bone loss with monthly oral ibandronate during adjuvant aromatase inhibitor therapy for breast cancer. *Clin Cancer Res.* 2008;14:6336-6342.

52. Van Poznak C, Hannon RA, Mackey JR, et al. Prevention of aromatase inhibitor-induced bone loss using risedronate: the SABRE trial. *J Clin Oncol.* 2010;28:967-975.

53. Brufsky AM, Harker WG, Beck JT, et al. Final 5-year results of Z-FAST trial: adjuvant zoledronic acid maintains bone mass in postmenopausal breast cancer patients receiving letrozole. *Cancer.* 2012;118:1192-1201.

54. Ellis GK, Bone HG, Chlebowski R, et al. Randomized trial of denosumab in patients receiving adjuvant aromatase inhibitors for nonmetastatic breast cancer. *J Clin Oncol.* 2008;26:4875-4882.

55. Smith MR, Eastham J, Gleason DM, Shasha D, Tchekmedyian S, Zinner N. Randomized controlled trial of zoledronic acid to prevent bone loss in men receiving androgen deprivation therapy for nonmetastatic prostate cancer. *J Urol.* 2003;169:2008-2012.

11

56. Smith MR, Egerdie B, Hernandez Toriz N, et al. Denosumab in men receiving androgen-deprivation therapy for prostate cancer. *N Engl J Med.* 2009;361:745-755.

57. Smith MR, Morton RA, Barnette KG, et al. Toremifene to reduce fracture risk in men receiving androgen deprivation therapy for prostate cancer. *J Urol.* 2010;184:1316-1321.

58. Andress DL, Ozuna J, Tirschwell D, et al. Antiepileptic drug-induced bone loss in young male patients who have seizures. *Arch Neurol.* 2002;59:781-786.

59. Ensrud KE, Walczak TS, Blackwell T, Ensrud ER, Bowman PJ, Stone KL. Antiepileptic drug use increases rates of bone loss in older women: a prospective study. *Neurology.* 2004;62:2051-2057.

60. Zhou C, Assem M, Tay JC, et al. Steroid and xenobiotic receptor and vitamin D receptor crosstalk mediates CYP24 expression and drug-induced osteomalacia. *J Clin Invest.* 2006;116:1703-1712.

61. Pascussi JM, Robert A, Nguyen M, et al. Possible involvement of pregnane X receptor-enhanced CYP24 expression in drug-induced osteomalacia. *J Clin Invest.* 2005;115:177-186.

62. Feldkamp J, Becker A, Witte OW, Scharff D, Scherbaum WA. Long-term anticonvulsant therapy leads to low bone mineral density–evidence for direct drug effects of phenytoin and carbamazepine on human osteoblast-like cells. *Exp Clin Endocrinol Diabetes.* 2000;108:37-43.

63. Wu S, Legido A, De Luca F. Effects of valproic acid on longitudinal bone growth. *J Child Neurol.* 2004;19:26-30.

64. Petty SJ, Wilding H, Wark JD. Osteoporosis associated with epilepsy and the use of anti-epileptics. A review. *Curr Osteoporos Rep.* 2016;14(2):54-65.

65. Dahlman TC, Sjoberg HE, Ringertz H. Bone mineral density during long-term prophylaxis with heparin in pregnancy. *Am J Obstet Gynecol.* 1994;170:1315-1320.

66. Barbour LA, Kick SD, Steiner JF, et al. A prospective study of heparin-induced osteoporosis in pregnancy using bone densitometry. *Am J Obstet Gynecol.* 1994;170:862-869.

67. Watt NB, Bilezikian JP, Usiskin K, et al. Effects of canagliflozin on fracture risk in patient with type 2 diabetes mellitus. *J Clin Endocrinol Metab.* 2016;10:157-166.

12 Abbreviations/Acronyms

1,25-(OH)$_2$D$_3$	1,25-dihydroxyvitamin D$_3$
25-(OH)$_2$D	1,25-dihydroxyvitamin D$_2$
AACE	American Association of Clinical Endocrinologists
ACF	autocorrelation function
ADT	androgen deprivation therapy
AEDs	anti-epileptic drugs
AHRQ	The Agency for Healthcare Research and Quality
AI	aromatase inhibitor
AP	anterior-posterior
APC	adenomatosis polyposis coli
ATAC	Arimidex, Tamoxifen, Alone or in Combination [trial]
AWHA	Adult Women's Health Alliance
BCF	bias correction factor
BGP	bone GLA-protein
BMC	bone mineral content
BMD	bone mineral density
BMI	body mass index
BMU	basic multicellular unit
BONE	Oral Ibandronate Osteoporosis Vertebral Fracture Trial in North America and Europe [study]
BSAP	bone-specific alkaline phosphatase
BSIt	torsional bone strength index
BTM	bone turnover markers
BUA	broadband ultrasound attenuation
C-cells	parafollicular cells
Ca	calcium
cAMP	cyclic adenosine monophosphate
CAROC	Canadian Association of Radiologist and Osteoporosis Canada
CaSR	calcium sensing receptor
CEE	conjugated equine estrogen

CI	confidence interval
CMS	Centers for Medicare & Medicaid Services
CNS	central nervous system
CoA	cortical bone area
COMT	catechol-0-methyltransferase
CORE	Continuing Outcomes Relevant to Evista [study]
CRF	clinical risk factor
CSF	colony-stimulating factor
c-src	cellular sarcoma
CT	computed tomography
CTX	C-terminal cross-linking telopeptide
CTx	C-carboxytelopeptide
CTX-MMP	C-terminal cross-linking telopeptide of type 1 collagen generated by metalloproteinases
CV	coefficient of variation
CVD	cardiovascular disease
DALY	disability and life-years
DHEA	dehydroepiandrosterone
DHEAS	dehydroepiandrosterone sulphate
DHT	dihydrotestosterone
DLX	distal-less homeobox
DIPART	Vitamin D Individual Patient Analysis of Randomised Trials
DKK1	dickkopf-1
DPD	deoxypyridinoline
dPyr	deoxypyridinoline
DVT	deep vein thrombosis
DXA	dual-energy x-ray absorptiometry
E/A	estrogen/androgen
E_1	estrone
E_2	estradiol
ER	estrogen receptor
ESCEO	European Society for Clinical and Economic Aspects of Osteoporosis and Osteoarthritis
ESE	esterified estrogen
ET	estrogen therapy
FAK	focal adhesion kinase
FDA	Food and Drug Administration
FGF	fibroblast growth factor
FIT	Fracture Intervention Trial [study]

FLEX	Fracture Intervention Trial Long-Term Extension [study]
FRAX	fracture risk assessment tool
FRC	Fracture Risk Calculator
FREE	Efficacy and safety of balloon kyphoplasty compared with non-surgical care for vertebral compression fracture [trial]
FREEDOM	Fracture Reduction Evaluation of Denosumab in Osteoporosis Every 6 Months [study]
FSH	follicle-stimulating hormone
GC	glucocorticoid
GGP	geranylgeranyl pyrophosphate
GFR	glomerular filtration rate
GH	growth hormone
GI	gastrointestinal
GIOP	glucocorticoid-induced osteoporosis
GM-CSF	granulocyte-macrophage colony-stimulating factor
GnRH	gonadotropin-releasing hormone
GRH	gonadotropin-releasing hormone
GSK	glycogen synthase kinase 3
HAL	hip axis length
HCTZ	hydrochlorothiazide
HDL	high-density lipoprotein
HERS	Heart and Estrogen/Progestin Replacement Study
hGH	human growth hormone
HIP	Hip Intervention Program [study]
HORIZON	Health Outcomes and Reduced Incidence With Zoledronic Acid Once Yearly [study]
HRT	hormone replacement therapy
HS	half strength
HSD	hydroxysteroid
HT	hormone therapy
HVDRR	hereditary vitamin D-resistant rickets
ICE	intermittent cyclic etidronate
ICS	impaired contrast sensitivity
ICTP	carboxyterminal telopeptide of type 1 collagen
IFCC	International Federation of Clinical Chemistry and Laboratory Medicine

12

IGF	insulin-like growth factor
IL	interleukin
IM	intramuscular
IOF	Internation Osteoporosis Foundation
iPTH	intact parathyroid hormone level
ISCD	International Society for Clinical Densitometry
IU	international units
IUD	intrauterine device
IV	intravenous
JNK	Jun kinase
Kg	kilogram
lb	pound
LDL	low-density lipoprotein
LIFT	Long-term Intervention on Fractures with Tibolone [study]
LRP	low-density lipoprotein receptor-related protein
LSC	least significant change
LT	lymphotoxin
m	meter
M-CSF	macrophage colony-stimulating factor
MeO-E	hydroxyestrogen monomethylether
MI	myocardial infarction
MMP	matrix metalloproteinase
MOBILE	Monthly Oral Ibandronate in Ladies [study]
MORE	Multiple Outcomes of Raloxifene Evaluation [study]
MOTION	Monthly Oral Therapy With Ibandronate for Osteoporosis Intervention [study]
MPa	megapascal
MPA	medroxyprogesterone acetate
MRI	magnetic resonance imagine
MSX2	Msh homeobox 2
NETA	norethindrone acetate
NFPP	Nijmegen Falls Prevention Program
NF-κB	nuclear factor kappa B
NHANES	National Health and Nutrition Examination Survey
NO	nitric oxide

NOF	National Osteoporosis Foundation
NORA	National Osteoporosis Risk Assessment
NTX	N-terminal
NTx	N-carboxytelopeptide
OH-E	hydroxyestrogen
ONJ	osteonecrosis of the jaw
OPG	osteoprotegerin
pDXA	oeripheral DXA
PG	prostaglandin
PI3K	phosphatidylinositol 3-kinase
P1CP	procollagen type I C-terminal peptide
P1NP	procollagen type I N-terminal peptide
PKA	protein kinase A
PKC	protein kinase C
PO	orally [by mouth]
PPARγ	peroxisome proliferator-activated receptor γ
PPI	proton pump inhibitors
pQCT	peripheral quantitative computed tomography
PRN	as needed
PROOF	Prevent Recurrence of Osteoporosis Fractures [study]
PTH	parathyroid hormone
PTH1R	PTH 1 receptor
Pyr	pyridinoline
QCT	quantitative computed tomography
QOL	Quality of Life
QUI	quantitative ultrasound index
QUS	quantitative ultrasound
RA	rheumatoid arthritis
RANK	receptor activator of NF-κB
RANKL	RANK ligand
RCT	randomized controlled trial
RDA	recommended daily allowance
REAL	Risedronate and Alendronate Cohort Study [study]
RM	repetition maximum
ROI	region of interest
RR	relative risk
RRR	relative risk reduction
RUNX2	Runt-related transcription factor 2

12

RXR	retinoid X receptor
SC	subcutaneous
SCT	salmon calcitonin
SD	standard deviation
SERMS	selective estrogen receptor modulators
SHBG	sex hormone binding globulin
SMA	Sequential Multiple Analysis
SOS	speed of sound through bone (ultrasound transit velocity)
SOTI	Spinal Osteoporosis Therapeutic Intervention [study]
SPA	single-photon absorptiometry
SSRIs	selective serotonin reuptake inhibitors
STAR	Study of Tamoxifen and Raloxifene [study]
SXA	single-energy x-ray absorptiometry
TGFα	transforming growth factor-alpha
TGFβ	transforming growth factor-beta
TH	total hip
TNF	tumor necrosis factor
TOP	Treatment of Osteoporosis With PTH [study]
TRACP5b	tartrate-resistant acid phosphatase 5b
TRAF	tumor necrosis factor receptor associated factor
TROPOS	Treatment of Peripheral Osteoporosis [study]
TSH	thyroid stimulating hormone
UCR	ultrasound critical angle reflectometry
UD	ultra distal
USDA	United States Department of Agriculture
USPSTF	United States Preventive Services Task Force
VDR	1,25-dihydroxyvitamin D receptor
VDRE	vitamin D response element
VFA	vertebral fracture assessment
VTE	venous thromboembolic disease
WBV	whole body vibration
WHI	Women's Health Initiative
WHO	World Health Organization
WNT	Wingless-type MMTV integration site

Note: Page numbers in *italics* indicate figures.
Page numbers followed by a "t" indicate tables.

Abaloparatide (PTHrP[1-34]), 181t, 234, 237-239. See also
  Parathyroid hormone (PTH).
 action mechanism, 237
 approved indications, 234, 237
 black box warning, 237
 contraindications and cautions, 238-239, 270
 dosage, 181t, 239
 efficacy, 238, *240-241*
 side effects, 238-239
Acidic environment, created by osteoclasts, 26, 259
ACTIVE trials, 238, *240-241*
Activities of daily living, 140
Actonel. See *Risedronate.*
Adolescence
 bone mass in, 24, 46
 bone remodeling in, 24
Adrenal function tests, 88
Advanced glycation end products (AGEs), 270
Adynamic bone disease, 271
Age/aging. See also *Elderly persons.*
 bone loss, 43, *45*, 72, 267
 bone mass, 44
 bone remodeling, 23-24, *24*, *25*
 osteopenia and, *13*
 for osteoporosis screening, 107-108, 107t
 peak bone mass, 23, *24*, 44
Alcohol intake
 falls, risk of, 51
 osteoporosis/fracture risk and, 62t, 63, 86, 268
 recommendations, 280
Alendronate, 180t, 185-193. See also *Bisphosphonates.*
 approved indications, 180t, 185, 191
  for men, 185, 268
  prevention and treatment of GIOP, 276
 chemical structure, *184*
 discontinuation of treatment, 190-191, *190*

Alendronate *(continued)*
  dosage, 180t, 187-190, 191-193
    daily dosing, 187
    once-weekly dosing, 187-190
  efficacy, 180t, 185-187
    bone mineral density, 187-190, *188-189*
    fracture risk reduction, 180t, 187, *190*, *192*
    glucocorticoid-induced osteoporosis, 191, *192*, 276
  formulation with vitamin D, 192-193
  long-term use, "drug holiday" for, 206, 245
  side effects, 180t
Alendronate/cholecalciferol, 180t
Alkaline phosphatase, 23
  as bone formation biomarker, 128t, 129
  bone-specific (BSAP), 128t
Aluminum, 62t, 271
Amenorrhea, exercise-induced, 60t, 66
American Association of Clinical Endocrinology (AACE),
    osteoporosis screening recommendation, 107-108
Androgens
  age-related decrease in, 268
  androgen deprivation therapy, 285-286
  hypogonadal states, 60t
Anorexia nervosa, 60t, 65-66
Anterior uveitis, 210
Anticoagulants, 62t
Anticonvulsants, 62t, 67
Antiepileptic drugs, 269, 286
Antiresorptive agents, 179, 180t-181t, 183-233. See also
    specific drug classes and agents.
  approved indications, 179, 180t-181t
  combinations not recommended, 182-183
  drug classes, 179, 180t-181t
    bisphosphonates, 180t, 183-210
    calcitonin, 181t, 227-229
    cathepsin K inhibitor (odanacatib), *260*, 261
    other drugs, 181t
    postmenopausal hormone replacement therapy, 179,
      231-233
    RANKL inhibitor (denosumab), 181t, 214-227
    selective estrogen receptor modulators, 181t, 210-214
    tyrosine src kinase inhibitor (saracatinib), *260*, 261

Antiresorptive agents *(continued)*
 efficacy, 181t
 novel therapies and targets, 260-261, *260*
 PTH in combination with or following, 239-243, *242, 243*
Antitransglutaminase antibodies, 86
Appendicular skeleton, 19, *20*
 cortical bone in, 22
Arimidex, 281
Aromatase inhibitors, 62t, 281-285
Arthralgias, 210
Arthritis, 269
Asian women, osteoporosis risk and, 11, 59
Asthma, 268-269
Astronauts, 37
Athletes
 amenorrhea in, 60t, 66
 female athletic triad, 66
Atrial fibrillation, 207
Autoimmune diseases, 61t
Axial skeleton, 19, *20*
 trabecular bone in, 22

Back pain, 59, 73, 137. See also *Pain.*
 causes of, 73, 139
 chronic, 137
Balance. See also *Falls.*
 falls prevention and, 140-141
 leg length disparity and, 73, *76-77*
 training and physical therapy for, 139-140
Balicatib, 261
Barbiturates, 62t
Basic multicellular unit (BMU), 31
BGP (bone GLA-protein). See *Osteocalcin.*
Biochemical markers of bone remodeling, 127-135, 128t
 bone formation, 128t, 129
 bone resorption, 128t, 129-131, *130*
Bisphosphonates, 180t, 183-210. See also *Antiresorptive agents; specific agents.*
 absorption of, 185
 action mechanisms, 184-185, *186*
 approved indications, 180t, 280
 cautions and contraindications, 203, 207, 273

13

Bisphosphonates *(continued)*
  chemical structures, *184*
  in children, 210
  dosage, 180t
  efficacy, 180t, 185-210, 285
  as first-line treatment, 182
  generations of
    first generation, 183
    second generation, 183
    third generation, 184
  long-term use, 133, 244-245
    "drug holiday" for, 133, 206, 245
  pharmacology, 183-185, *184*
  side effects and safety issues, 15, 180t, 204-210, 244-245
    anterior uveitis, 210
    arthralgias, 210
    atrial fibrillation, 207
    atypical femoral fractures, 206, *208-209*, 245
    fracture healing, 209
    gastrointestinal effects, 204-205
    hypocalcaemia, 210
    osteonecrosis of the jaw (ONJ), 205-206, *205*, 245
    post infusion acute phase reactions, 207
    renal impairment, 207, 273
    suppression of bone remodeling, 133
  specific agents, 180t
Blood pressure, 72-73
BMD. See *Bone mineral density.*
BMI. See *Body mass index.*
Body mass index (BMI), 72-73
  osteoporosis risk and, 14, 63
Body weight, 62t, 72-73
Bone, 19-42. See also *Cortical bone; Trabecular bone; and
  other bone entries.*
  anatomical structure, 19, *20*
  architectural structure, 19-22, *21*
  cells. See *Osteoblasts; Osteoclasts; Osteocytes.*
  chemical structure, 22-23
  cortical bone, 19-22, *21*
  embryological structure, 19
  functions of, 19
  intramembranous vs endochondral bone, 19

Bone *(continued)*
  mineral composition of, 149
  structure of, 19-23
  trabecular bone, 22, 43-44
Bone densitometry. See *DXA.*
Bone density, 81
Bone formation, 23. See also *Bone remodeling.*
  biochemical markers of, 128t, 129
  in bone remodeling cycle, *33,* 34-35
  inadequate, 48-49. See also *Osteopenia.*
  stimulants of, 179, 181t, 245. See also *Androgens;*
      Parathyroid hormone.
Bone fragility, 11
Bone GLA-protein. See *Osteocalcin.*
Bone homeostasis, 36, 271
Bone loss. See also *Bone remodeling; Risk factors for*
    osteoporosis.
  accelerated, 47-48
  aromatase inhibitors and, 281-285
  in astronauts, 37
  asymptomatic, 14
  cancer chemotherapy and, 281, *284*
  in children, 268-270
  chronic kidney disease and, 271-273
  drugs and, 273-287
  glucocorticoids and, 49, 274, *275,* 276
  hyperparathyroidism and, 271-273, *272*
  hyperprolactinemia and, 66
  immunosuppressive therapy and, 280-281
  medications and, 268-269, 273-287
  postmenopausal, 43
  risk factors for, 60t-62t
  secondary, 267
  thyroid hormones and, 36
Bone marrow, 35
Bone mass
  age and, 44
  antiresorptive agents and, 181t, 227-229
  in children and adolescents, 268-270
  exercise and, 46-47, 137-138
  female athletic triad and, 66
  fracture risk and, 89-90

13

Bone mass *(continued)*
  gynecologic factors in, 63-65t
  lifestyle and, 63
  medications associated with, 13-14, 59, 67
    glucocorticoids, *32*, 48, 49, 268-269, 274
  peak
    achieving before menopause, 137
    age at, 23, *24*, 63
    failure to achieve, 44-47
    genetics and, 46, 63, 268
  reference values, 83, 89
  reporting of, 88-89
  T-scores vs Z-scores, 82t, 83
Bone mass measurement. See also *DXA.*
  osteoporosis screening, age for, 107-108, 107t
  technology/techniques, 14
Bone matrix
  constituents/synthesis, 26, *29*
  mineral to matrix ratio, 50
Bone metabolism, endocrine factors in, 35-36
Bone mineral density (BMD), 68-69, 88-90. See also *Bone mass; DXA; Fracture risk.*
  bone strength and, 89
  exercise and, 127-128
  loss with age, 267
  measured by DXA, 14, 68-69, 70t
  medications and, 274
  in men, 86, 267-268
  as predictive of fracture risk, 14, 59, 89-90
  sites recommended for, 83
  T-scores, 81-83, 82t
Bone morphogenetic proteins, 28
Bone quality, 49-50, 81
Bone remodeling, 23-35. See also *Bone formation; Bone resorption.*
  acidic environment for, 26
  age and gender in, 23-24, *24*, *25*
  basic multicellular unit (BMU) in, 31, 34
  biochemical markers of, 127-135, 128t
    bone formation, 128t, 129
    bone resorption, 128t, 129-131

Bone remodeling *(continued)*
  bone remodeling cycle, 31-35, *33*
    activation, 32-34, *33*
    osteoblast activation and osteoid formation, *33*, 34-35
    osteoclast activation and resorption, *33*, 34, 259-260, *260*
    quiescence, 35
  bone resorption in, 44, 260
  cells regulating, 24-31
  endocrine factors in, 35-36
  exercise and, 36-37
  mechanical stress and, 36-37
  osteoblasts in, 26-31, *33*, 34-35, 127, 259, 262, *263*
  osteoclasts in, 24-26, *27*, *33*, 34, 127, 259-261, *260*
  suppression of, 127, 133
Bone resorption, 44, 260. See also *Antiresorptive agents;*
  Bone loss.
  accelerated, 47-48
  antiresorptive agents, 179, 180t-181t, 260-261
  cathepsin K in, 259, *260*, 261
  markers of, 128t, 129-131, *130*
Bone-specific alkaline phosphatase (BSAP), 128t
BONE study (Oral Ibandronate), 196
Bone strength
  BMD and, 89
  changes with age, *25*
Bone turnover markers (BTM), 127-135, 128t
  in clinical practice, 131-133
  formation markers, 128t
  lack of standardized testing, 131-132
  in monitoring osteoporosis therapy, 132-133
  as predictors of fracture risk, 127, 132
  resorption markers, 128t, 129-131, *130*
Boniva. See *Ibandronate.*
Breast cancer, 281-285
  aromatase inhibitors and, 281-285
  aromatase inhibitors in therapy for, 281
  raloxifene, reduction of breast cancer risk, 210, 212
  risk, 231-233, *232*
  tibolone and, 214

C-carboxytelopeptide (CTX), 128t, *130*, 131
C-telopeptide, *130*, 217, 219

13

Caffeine intake, 63
Calcaneus, QUS of, 106, 110, 112
Calcilytic drugs, 265
Calcitonin, 181t, 227-229
  action mechanisms, 36, 227
  dosage and administration, 229
  efficacy, 181t, 227-228
    intranasal, 228
    parenteral, 227-228
  indications for, 181t
  salmon calcitonin (SCT), 181t, 227
  side effects, 181t, 228
Calcium, 149-162. See also *Vitamin D.*
  absorption of, 156
    aging and, 163
  calcium calculator, 149, *152-155*
  deficiency, 46-47
  Dietary Reference Intakes for, 149, 150t-151t
    for postmenopausal women, 149
  dietary sources, 149, 158
    milk and dairy products, 160
  food label, 156, *157*
  fracture reduction and, 158-160, *159*
  intake, 156-158
    cardiovascular concerns, 160-162
    daily need for, 156
    dietary reference guidelines, 150t-151t
    low, as risk factor for osteoporosis, 60t, 63
    necessary for efficacy of anti-osteoporosis medications, 15
    recommended daily, 150t-151t, 158, 160
      in special populations, 269, 270, 276-280, 281-285, 286
    supplementation for, 63, 158
  malabsorption of, 67
  measurements of, in diagnosis, 86, 87t
  parathyroid hormone (PTH) and, 262, 265
  percentage in skeleton and hydroxyapatite, 149
  supplementary, 63, 158
    bioavailability of, 158
    calcium-fortified beverages, 158
    recommendations on, 158, 160
    side effects and concerns, 160-162
  vitamin D necessity for absorption of, 156

Calcium-sensing receptor (CaSR), 262, *263*, 264-265
Canagliflozin, 287
Cancellous bone. See *Trabecular bone.*
Cancer
  breast, 231-233, *232*, 281-285
  chemotherapy, 269, 281, *284*
  in children/adolescents, 269
  disability from, 13
  prostate, 228, 268, 285
CANVAS trial, 287
Cardiovascular disease (CVD)
  calcium supplementation and, 160-162
  denosumab and, 220
  PTH and, 246, *272*
  raloxifene and, 210, 212
  strontium and, 231
  thiazolidinediones and, 280
Caspase system, bisphosphonates and, 185, *186*
CaSR. See *Calcium-sensing receptor.*
Cathepsin K, 26, 259, *260*, 261
  inhibitor of (odanacatib), *260*, 261
Caucasian women, osteoporosis risk and, 11, 59
Celiac disease, 67, 86, 268
Centers for Medicare & Medicaid Services (CMS),
    108-109, 109t
Central nervous system disorders
  falls and, 51
  osteoporosis/fracture risk and, 61t
Chemotherapy, 62t, 281, *284*
Chief cells, 35
Childbirths, 64
Children, 268-270
  bone modeling in, 23
Chronic kidney disease (CKD), 271-273, *272*
Chronic kidney disease-mineral and bone disorder
    (CKD-MBD), 271
Cinacalcet, 273
Clinical evaluation. See *Diagnosis of osteoporosis.*
Clodronate, 183, *184*, 203
Collagen, 22, 49-50, 127, 270
  cathepsin K and, 261
  cross-links, 50, 128t, 129-131

13

Collagen *(continued)*
  fractures and, 49-50
  procollagen I terminal peptides, 128t, 129, *130*
CORE (Continuing Outcomes Relevant to Evista), 211-212
Cortical bone, 19-22, *21*
  loss of, 44, *45*
  percentage in different bones, *20*, 22
Corticosteroids. See *Glucocorticoids.*
CTX (C-terminal cross-linking telopeptide), 128t, *130*, 131, 219
Cushing's disease, 48, 61t, 88, 268
Cyclosporine, 62t

Daily living, activities of, 140
DALYs (disability and life-years lost), 11-13, *12*
Dapagliflozin, 287
DATA study, 220-225, *222-223*, *224*, *226*
Definition of osteoporosis, 81-83, 82t
Denosumab (RANKL inhibitor), 181t, 214-227
  action mechanism, 214-215, *216*, 260, *260*
  approved indications, 181t, 214, 280
  in CKD, 273
  DATA study, 220-225, *222-223*, *224*, *226*
  discontinuing treatment, 220-225, *222-223*, *224*, *226*
  dosage and administration, 181t, 225-227
  efficacy, 181t, 215-220
    bone mineral density, 215-220, 285
    fracture risk reduction, 215-220, *217*, 218t
  FREEDOM trial, 215-220, *217*, 218t
  indications for, 260
    androgen deprivation therapy, 285
    in men, 268
    as second-line treatment, 182
  long-term therapy, 245
    drug "holiday" NOT recommended, 245
  side effects, 181t, 220
Densitometry. See *DXA.*
Dental hygiene, 205-206
Deoxypyridinoline (DPD), 128t, *130*, 131
DEXA. See *DXA.*
Diabetes, 270
  as risk factor, 61t

Diagnosis of osteoporosis, 59-135
  after first clinical fracture, 14
  assessment tools, 109-115
  biochemical markers of bone remodeling, 127-135
    in clinical practice, 131-133
  bone densitometry, 14, 49, 88-106. See also *DXA.*
  bone mass, 89-90
    reporting and reference values, 88-89
  bone mineral density (BMD)
    DXA measurement of, 14, 68-69, 88-106
    T-scores, 81-83, 82t, 88-89
  definition of osteoporosis, 81-83, 82t
  DXA, 88-106
    interpretation of, 90-106
    screening and retesting, 106-110
    sites recommended for, 83, 90, *92-97*
  fracture risk assessment tools, 109-115
  fracture types, 84-86, *85*
  fragility fractures, 84-86, *85*
  FRAX as risk assessment tool, 14, 68-71, *69*, 70t-71t, 102
  history, 59, 60t-62t
  musculoskeletal examination, 73, *76-77*
  patient evaluation, 59
  physical examination, 72-73, 74t
    leg-length discrepancies, 73, *76-77*
  risk factors, 63-68
    eating disorders, 65-66
    endocrinopathies, 61t, 66
    fall risk factors, 67-68
    gastrointestinal diseases, 61t, 67
    genetics, 60t, 63
    gynecologic risk factors, 63-65
    lifestyle risk factors, 63
    medications, 62t, 67
    modifiable risk factors, 63
  screening and retesting, 106-110
  secondary causes of osteoporosis, 86-88
    laboratory tests for, 87t
  T-scores and Z-scores, 81-83, 82t, 88-89
  vertebral fracture assessment (VFA), 95, 114-115,
    116-117, 118t, *120-121*
Dickkopf-1. See *DKK1.*

13

Diet, 63, 149
  calcium in, 149-162
    sources of, 149
  vitamin D in, 162-169
    sources of, 163
Disability, 11-13, *12*
  disability and life-years (DALYs) lost, 11-13, *12*
Dizziness, 51, 68
DKK1 (dickkopf-1), 31, 262, *263*, 264
  antibody against (BHQ 880), *263*, 264
Dorsal kyphosis, 73
Drug therapy. See *Pharmacologic treatment.*
Drugs that increase fracture risk, 273-287. See also
    Medications.
Dual-energy x-ray absorptiometry. See *DXA.*
DXA (dual-energy x-ray absorptiometry), 14, 49, 81, 88-106
  advantages of, 88
  best practices for, 104, 105t
  fracture risk assessment with, 89-90
  indications for, 88, 106-110
    from CMS, 108-109, 109t
  interpretation of, 90-106, 105t
    assessment of change, 103-104
    certification for, 91
    comparisons with other scanners, 103-104
    forearm analysis, 103
    general analysis, 91
    hip analysis, 96-102
    lumbar spine analysis, 91-96
    patient information sheet, *98-101*
    quality assurance for, 104
    reference values, 89
  in pediatrics, 89
  peripheral DXA, 106-107
  quality of, 104, 105t
  reference values, 89
  reporting of, 88-89, 106
  screening recommendations, 106-110, 107t, 109t
  screening tests compared, 106-107
  sites recommended for, 83, 90, *92-97*
    forearm, 90, *96-97*
    hip, 90, *94-95*
    spine, 90, *92-93*

DXA (dual-energy x-ray absorptiometry) *(continued)*
  T-scores, 70t, 81-83, 82t, 88-89
  Z-scores, 81-83, 88-89

Eating disorders, osteoporosis/fracture risk and, 60t, 65-66
Elderly persons. See also *Age/aging.*
  falls
    prevention programs, 140-141
    risk of, 50-51, *52-53*, 67-68
  fractures in, morbidity and, 11
  walking speed and falls in, *52-53*
Empagliflozin, 287
Endochondral bone, 19
Endocrine factors in bone metabolism, 35-36, 61t, 66
Endosteum, 21, *21*
Epilepsy, 269
Estrogen. See also *Hormone therapy.*
  bone metabolism and, 36
  deficiency, 43, 47, 48, 64
  osteoblasts/osteoclasts/osteocytes, effects on, 36, 47
  selective estrogen receptor modulators (SERMs), 181t,
    210-214
Ethnicity
  DEXA reference values, 83, 89
  osteoporosis risk and, 11, 59
  Z-scores, 89
Etidronate, 183, 203-204
  chemical structure, *184*
  dosage, 204
  not FDA approved in the United States, 203-204
  off label use, 204
EUROFORS, 239-243
Evista. See *Raloxifene.*
Exercise, 137-140
  in adolescents/teens, 46-47
  balance training, 139-140
  bone mass and, 46-47, 137-138
  fracture risk and, 49, 138
  high-impact, 137-138
  lack of, 46-47, 49, 60t
  osteoporosis exercise program, 138-140
  physical therapist and, 139, 140

13

Exercise *(continued)*
  for postmenopausal women, 138-139
  for premenopausal women, 137-138
  site-specific, 139-140
  strength training, 138-139
  walking, 138, 140
  weight-bearing, 138, 139

Falls, 60t, 67-68, 140-141
  balance and, 140-141
  eliminating, 51
  factors in, 50-51, 67-68
    central nervous system disorders, 51
    dizziness, 51, 68
    medications, 51
    muscle mass and strength, 50
    soft tissue, 51
    visual impairment, 68
    walking speed, *52-53*
  fractures and, 50-51
    vitamin D and, 51, 168-169, *170*
  prevention of, 140-141
  vitamin D and, 51, 169
Family history, 59. See also *Genetic factors.*
Female athletic triad, 66
Femoral fractures. See also *Hip fractures.*
  atypical, bisphosphonates and, 206, *208-209*, 245
Femoral neck
  bone composition of, *20*, 22
  DXA of, 96-102
Femur, 22. See also *Femoral entries.*
Fibroblast growth factor-23 (FGF-23), 31
FIT (Fracture Intervention Trial), 190-191, *190*
FLEX study, 190-191, *190*
Forearm, bone densitometry of, 90, *96-97*, 103
Forteo. See *Parathyroid hormone.*
Fosamax. See *Alendronate.*
Fracture(s). See also *specific types of fractures.*
  cause of, 81
  distal radius, 11
  fragility fractures, 84-86, *85*
  FRAX (fracture risk assessment tool), 14, 68-71, *69*,
    70t-71t, 102

Fracture(s) *(continued)*
  hip, 11, 84
  mortality from, 11
  osteoporotic
    annual direct costs from, 13
    common sites of, *20*
  previous history of, 59, 70t, 84, *85*
  reduction with calcium intake, 158-160, *159*
  risk of. See *Fracture risk.*
  sites of, 11, *20*
  vertebral, 11, 84, *85*
Fracture risk, 11. See also *DXA.*
  age as predictor of, 49
  assessment
    initial, 276, *277*
    reassessment, 276, *278-279*
  assessment tools, 109-115
    DXA, 89-90
    Fracture Risk Calculator, 73, 109
    FRAX, 14, 68-71, *69*, 70t-71t, 102, 109
    Garvan fracture risk calculator, 73, 110
    QCT, 112-114, *113*
    Qfracture, 110
    QUS, 110-112, *111*
    trabecular bone score, 115, *122*
    vertebral fracture assessment (VFA), 95, 114-115,
      116-117, 118t, *120-121*
    websites for, 109-110
  bone mass and, 43, 89-90
  bone turnover and, 127
  bone turnover markers and, 127, 132
  calcium intake and, 158-160, *159*
  exercise and, 49, 138
  falls and, 50-51
  five main factors in, 44-51, *46*
    accelerated bone loss, 47-48
    failure to achieve peak bone mass, 44-47
    inadequate bone formation, 48-49
    increased fall risk, 50-51
    poor bone quality, 49-50
  genetics and, 46, 60t
  hormonal factors, 36, 60t-61t

13

Fracture risk *(continued)*
  hyperthyroidism and, 36
  leg length disparity and, 73
  medications and, 62t, 67, 273-287
    androgen deprivation therapy, 285-286
    anti-epileptic drugs, 286
    aromatase inhibitors, 281-285
    cancer chemotherapy, 281, *284*
    glucocorticoids, 274-280
    heparin, 286
    proton pump inhibitors, 273
    selective serotonin inhibitors (SSRIs), 274
    SGLT2 inhibitors, 286-287
    thiazolidinediones, 280
    transplant anti-rejection mediations, 280-281
  osteoporosis and, 81
  previous fractures and, 59, 70t, 84, *85*
  reduction by pharmacologic agents, 180t-181t
  sedentary lifestyle and, 46-47, 49
  in special populations, 267-292
  vitamin D and, 168-169, *170*
Fragility fractures, 84-86, *85*
  pharmacologic treatment and prevention, 183
Fragility of bone, 11
Framingham Study, 161
FRAX (fracture risk assessment tool), 14, 68-71, *69*,
    70t-71t, 102, 109
  in DXA interpretation, 96, 102
  threshold/indication for pharmacologic therapy, 183
FREEDOM trial, 215-220, *217*, 218t
Frizzled, *30*, 31, 262, *263*

Gabapentin, 67
Garvan fracture risk calculator, 73, 110
Gastrointestinal diseases, 61t, 67
Gastrointestinal side effects, 204-205
Genetic factors
  in osteoporosis/fracture risk, 60t, 63
  peak bone mass and, 46, 63, 268
GIOP (glucocorticoid-induced osteoporosis).
    See *Glucocorticoids, osteoporosis induced by.*
GLA-protein. See *Osteocalcin.*

Glucocorticoids, *32*, 48, 49, 268-269, 274-280
  bone formation/bone loss and, 36, 48, 49, 268-269,
    274-280, *275*
  duration of treatment, 276
  excess, 36
  inhaled, 268-269, 274
  intra-articular, 274
  osteoporosis/fracture risk and, 48, 62t, 70t, 86, 274-280,
    275
    fracture risk assessments, 276, *277*, *278-279*
  osteoporosis induced by (GIOP), 274-280
    in children, 269
    pathophysiology of, *275*
    pharmacologic treatment recommendations, 280, *282-283*
    prevention and treatment, 191, *192*, 194, 276, *277*
    PTH and, 243-244
  recommendations for patients receiving, 276-280
Gluten-free diet, 67
GnRH, 62t
Growth factors, 48
Growth hormone, 48
GSK-37, 262
Gynecologic factors in osteoporosis, 63-65

Haversian system, 21, *21*
Heel. See *Calcaneus.*
Height, 72
Hematologic disorders, 61t
Heparin, 286
HERS study, 231
Hip
  DXA of, 90, *94-95*
    analysis, 96-102
  fractures of. See *Hip fractures.*
  walking programs and, 140
Hip fractures, 11, *20*, 84, 138, 141
  bisphosphonates and (femoral fractures), 206, *208-209*
  family history of, 59
  impact of, 11, 84t
  mortality associated with, 11
  reduced with mechanical hip protectors, 141, *142-143*
Hip Intervention Program (HIP) trial, 194

13

Hip protectors, mechanical, 141, *142-143*
History, family, 59
History, patient, 59, 60t-62t
HORIZON trials, 199-202, *200*, 201t
Hormonal factors
  in bone formation/remodeling, 35-36
  in osteoporosis/fracture risk, 60t-61t
Hormone therapy (HT), 179, 231-233
  for menopause, 63, 231-233
    indicated for early menopause, 233
  postmenopausal hormone replacement therapy, 179,
    231-233
    not approved for treatment of osteoporosis, 182
    side effects, 231-233
  risks of, 231-233
    risk/benefit analysis, 232, *232*
Hydroxyapatite, 22-23, 149
  dissolution of, 26
Hyperparathyroidism, 268, 271-273, *272*
  osteoporosis risk and, 61t
  secondary, 47
Hyperprolactinemia, 60t, 66
Hyperthyroidism, 36, 66
Hypocalcaemia, 210
Hypogonadal states, 60t, 86
Hysterectomy, 65

Ibandronate, 180t, 195-199. See also *Bisphosphonates.*
  approved indications, 180t, 195-196
  BONE study, 196
  chemical structure, *184*
  dosage and administration, 180t, 199
    intravenous treatment, 198
    oral treatment, 196-198
    oral vs intravenous, 198-199
  efficacy, 180t, 196-199
    bone mineral density, 196-198, *197*
    fracture risk reduction, 180t, 196
  MOBILE study, 196-198, *197*
  potency of, 195
  side effects, 180t, 204
Idiopathic osteoporosis, 43

Immunosuppressive therapy, 280-281
Inflammatory bowel disease, 269
Inflammatory cytokines, 48
Insulin-like growth factors (IGFs), 48
Integrins
  bisphosphonates and, 185
  osteoclast function and, 259, *260*
Interleukin-1 (IL-1), 26, *28*, 48
International Federation of Clinical Chemistry and
    Laboratory Medicine (IFCC), 131
Intracortical bone, 21, *21*
Intramembranous bone, 19
ISCD, criteria/recommendations for BMD testing, 90,
    107-108

Kidney disease, chronic, 271-273
Kidney stones, 162
Kyphoplasty, 143-146, *145*
Kyphosis, 139

Lactation, 64
  osteoporosis risk and, 64-65
LDL receptor-related proteins (LRP5/6), 262, *263*
Leg length disparities, 73, *76-77*
Levetiracetam, 67
Lifestyle, 46-47, 63
  modifications, 280
  osteoporosis/fracture risk and, 46-47, 49, 60t, 63
  risk factors, 63
  sedentary, 46-47, 49
Lipid levels, raloxifene and, 211
Low bone mass (osteopenia), *25*
  WHO definition of, 82t
  in women ages 50 and older, *13*
Lumbar spine. See also *Vertebrae.*
  bone mass in, *20*
    T-scores and Z-scores for, *93*
  DXA of, 90, 91-96, *92-93*

M-CSF (macrophage colony-stimulating factor), 26, *27*, 34,
    260
Macrophage colony-stimulating factor. See *M-CSF.*

Malabsorption, 61t, 67
Markers. See *Bone turnover markers*.
Marrow. See *Bone marrow*.
Matrix metalloproteinases, 26
Mechanical strength of bone. See *Bone strength*.
Mechanical stress and force, 36-37
Medicare/Medicaid services and follow-up testing,
    108-109, 109t
Medications
  bone loss and, 268-270, 273-287
  decline in bone associated with, 13-14, 59
  fall risk and, 51
  osteoporosis/fracture risk and, 62t, 67, 273-287
    androgen deprivation therapy, 285-286
    anti-epileptic drugs, 286
    aromatase inhibitors, 281-285
    cancer chemotherapy, 281, *284*
    glucocorticoids, 268-269, 274-280
    heparin, 286
    proton pump inhibitors, 273
    selective serotonin inhibitors (SSRIs), 274
    SGLT2 inhibitors, 286-287
    thiazolidinediones, 280
    transplant anti-rejection mediations, 280-281
Medroxyprogesterone (depo-medroxyprogesterone), 62t
Men, 267-268
  causes of low BMD in, 86, 267-268
  DXA screening in, 108, 109
  osteoporosis in, 267-268
    approved pharmacologic agents for, 268
Menarche, late onset, bone mass and, 64
Menopause, 63, 65
  bone loss after, 43, 44, 65
  early/surgical, 60t, 63, 233
  estrogen deficiency, 43, 47
  hormone replacement therapy and, 63, 231-233
  osteoporosis and, 43, 65
Menstruation
  amenorrhea, exercise-induced, 60t, 66
  history of, 64
  late menarche, 64
Metabolic disorders, 61t

Microcrack repair, *33*

Microfractures, 49

MK-5442, *263*, 265

MOBILE (Monthly Oral Ibandronate in Ladies) study, 196-198, *197*

MORE (Multiple Outcomes of Raloxifene Evaluation), 211

Muscle mass, age-related loss of, 50

Muscle strength, vitamin D and, 169, *172-173*

Musculoskeletal examination, 73, 74t, *76-77*

N-carboxytelopeptide (NTx), 128t, *130*

National Osteoporosis Foundation (NOF)
  on costs of osteoporotic fractures, 13
  osteoporosis screening recommendation, 107-108

NF-κB ligand, 26, *27*, 260, *260*

NHANES (National Health and Nutrition Examination Survey), 83, 89, 156-157

Nitric oxide, 37

NOF. See *National Osteoporosis Foundation.*

Non-collagenous proteins, 22-23

Nonpharmacologic therapy, 137-148
  exercise and physical therapy, 137-140
  fall prevention, 140-141
  hip protectors, 141, *142-143*
  surgical intervention, challenges of, 146
  vertebral stabilization, 142-146, *144*, *145*

NTX (N-terminal cross-linking telopeptide), 128t, *130*

Nurse's Health Study, 161

Nutrition, 63. See also *Diet.*

Odanacatib, *260*, 261

Older persons. See *Elderly persons.*

OPG. See *Osteoprotegerin.*

Oral contraceptives, 269

Oral hygiene, 205-206

Orthostatic hypotension, 68, 72-73

Osteoblasts, 26-31, 262-265
  bone formation biomarkers of, 28, 127
  bone remodeling and, 26-31, *33*, 34-35, 259
  differentiation of, 26-31, *29*, 262, *263*
  estrogen effects on, 47
  glucocorticoids and, 49, 274, *275*

13

Osteoblasts *(continued)*
  mechanical force and, 37
  novel therapeutic targets, 259, 262-265, *263*
  parathyroid hormone (PTH) and, 28, 234, 262, *263*
  physiology and therapeutic targets, 259, 262-265, *263*
  stimulators and inhibitors of, *32*
  vitamin D and, 163
  Wnt/β-catenin signaling pathway and, 28, *30*, 34, 37,
    262-264, *263*
Osteocalcin (bone GLA-protein, BGP), 23, 34, 128t, 129
Osteoclasts, 24-26, 259-261
  acidic environment created by, 26, 259
  in bone loss, 44
  bone remodeling and, 24-26, *27*, *33*, 34, 127, 259
  calcitonin and, 227
  cathepsin K and, 259, 261
  differentiation of, 26, *27*, 259-260
  estrogen effects on, 37, 47
  functions of, 24-26
  mechanical force and, 37
  novel therapeutic targets, 259-261, *260*
  parathyroid hormone and, 26, 234
  physiology and therapeutic targets, 259-261, *260*
  ruffled border, 26, *28*, 34
  stimulators and inhibitors of, 26, *28*
  tyrosine src-kinase and, 261
Osteocytes, 31, *33*
  apoptosis, bisphosphonates and, 185
  mechanical loading and, 31
Osteoid, *33*, 34-35
Osteomalacia, 271
Osteonecrosis of the jaw (ONJ), 205-206, *205*, 245
Osteopenia, *25*
  prevalence in women ages 50 and older, *13*
Osteopontin, 23, 34
Osteoporosis
  characteristics of, *25*
  in children, 268-270
  definition of, 81-83, 82t
  diagnosis of, 59-135
  impact of, 11-17, 137
  pathogenesis of, 43-57

Osteoporosis *(continued)*
  prevalence in women ages 50 and older, 13-14, *13*
  prevention and treatment, 137-257
  primary vs secondary, 43, 86-88
  risk. See *Risk factors for osteoporosis.*
  societal burden of, 11-17
  in special populations, 267-292
Osteoprotegerin (OPG), 26, 34, 47
  RANKL:OPG ratio, 26
Osteosarcoma
  abaloparatide and, 270
  parathyroid hormone and, 237
  teriparatide and, 237, 270

Paget's disease, 50, 238
  bisphosphonates for, 203
Pain
  back pain, 59, 73
  relief with vertebroplasty, 143
  of spinal fractures, 137
Pamidronate, 183, 203
Parafollicular cells, 36
Parathyroid hormone (PTH), 35, 181t, 233-244. See also
    Abaloparatide; Hyperparathyroidism; Teriparatide.
  action mechanisms, 35, 234
  agents, 181t, 234
    abaloparatide (PTHrP[1-34]), 181t, 234, 237-239
    as recombinant human PTH, 234, 235
    teriparatide (rhPTH[1-34]), 181t, 234, 235-237
  analogues, 181t, 233-244
  approved indications, 181t
  biologic basis for anabolic effect, 233-234
  black box warning for teriparatide, 235, 237
  bone turnover and, *272*
  calcium level, maintenance of, 262, 265
  calcium-sensing receptor (CaSR) and, 262, *263*, 264-265
  in CKD, *272*
  in combination with antiresorptive therapy, 239-243, *242*,
    243
  cost of, 182, 246
  dosage, formulations, and use, 181t
  duration of therapy, 246

13

Parathyroid hormone (PTH) *(continued)*
  efficacy, 181t, 235, 238, 246
    bone mineral density, 235, 236t
    fracture risk reduction, 235, *236*, 236t, 238, *240-241*, 244, *245*
  glucocorticoid-induced osteoporosis and, 243-244
  intact PTH (iPTH), 271-273
  measurements of, 86
  osteoblasts and osteoclasts, effects on, 26, 28, *32*, 234, 262, *263*
  receptors, 35, 234, 237
  side effects and safety concerns, 181t, 235-239
    osteosarcoma, 237-238
  trabecular connectivity and, 244, *245*
  vitamin D and, 35, 47
Parenteral nutrition, 62t
Parity, 64
Pathogenesis of osteoporosis, 43-57
  cortical bone loss, 44, *45*
  main factors in, 44-51, *46*
  trabecular bone loss, 43-44, *45*
Patient education, 15
Peak bone mass, 23, *24*, 44-47, 63
Periosteum, 21, *21*
Peripheral sites, testing of, 106-107
Pharmacologic treatment, 179-266. See also *specific agents.*
  antiresorptive agents, 179, 180t-181t, 183-233
    combinations not recommended, 182-183
  bisphosphonates, 180t, 183-210
  bone formation stimulants, 179, 181t, 245
  calcitonin, 181t, 227-229
  drug classes, 179, 180t-181t
  efficacy of, 14, 180t-181t
    concurrent calcium and vitamin D necessary, 15
    fracture risk reduction, 180t-181t, 182
  evolving pathways and therapeutic targets, 259-266, *260*, *263*
    calcium-sensing receptor (CaSR), 262, *263*, 264-265
    cathepsin K, 259, *260*, 261
    DKK1, 262, *263*, 264
    sclerostin, 262-264, *263*
    tyrosine src-kinase, *260*, 261

Pharmacologic treatment *(continued)*
  general guidelines for, 182-183
  for glucocorticoid-induced osteoporosis (GIOP), 280,
    282-283
  hormone replacement therapy, 182-183, 231-233
  indications for, 180t-181t, 183
  long-term treatment, current perspective, 244-246
  novel agents, 259-266, *260, 263*
  parathyroid hormone/PTH analogues, 181t, 233-244
  RANKL inhibitor (denosumab), 181t, 214-227
  risk/benefit ratio of, 15
  safety of, 14-15, 244-245
  selective estrogen receptor modulators, 181t, 210-214
  strontium ranelate, 181t, 229-231
Physical activity. See *Exercise.*
Physical examination, 72-73, 74t
Physical therapy, 139-140
Physiology of bone, 19-42
PICP (procollagen type I C-terminal peptide), 128t, 129,
  130
PINP (procollagen type I N-terminal peptide), 128t, 129,
  130, 219
Pioglitazone, 62t
Prednisone, 48, 243
Pregnancy
  medications contraindicated in, 203
  osteoporosis risk and, 64-65
Prevention and treatment, 137-266. See also *specific
  therapies and agents.*
  bone turnover markers in monitoring treatment, 132-133
  calcium, 149-162
  evolving pathways and therapeutic targets, 259-266
  exercise and physical therapy, 137-140
  hip protectors, 141, *142-143*
  long-term treatment, current perspective, 244-246
  nonpharmacologic therapy, 137-148
  pharmacologic agents, 179-266
    evolving agents and therapeutic targets, 259-266, *260,
      263*
  vertebral stabilization, 142-146, *144, 145*
  vitamin D, 162-169
Primary osteoporosis, 43

13

Procollagen I terminal peptides, 128t, 129, *130*
Prostaglandins, *32*, 37
Prostate cancer, 228, 268, 285
Proton pump inhibitors, 62t, 273
PTH. See *Parathyroid hormone.*
Pyridinium cross-links, 128t, 129-131, *130*
Pyridinoline, 128t, *130*, 131

QCT (quantitative computed tomography), 112-114, *113*
Quality of life, impact of osteoporosis on, 11-17, 137
Quantitative bone ultrasound (QUS), 106-107, 110-112, *111*
Quantitative computed tomography (QCT), 112-114, *113*
QUS. See *Quantitative bone ultrasound.*

Race. See *Ethnicity.*
Radius, 22
  distal, fractures in, 11
Raloxifene, 181t, 210-212
  action mechanism, 210
  approved indications, 181t, 210, 280
    as second-line treatment, 182
  dosage, 181t, 212
  efficacy, 211-212
  side effects, 181t, 212
  systemic beneficial effects, 210-211
RANK-RANKL, 26, *27*, 34, 48, 260
  bisphosphonates and, 185
  in bone remodeling, 34, 35, 260, *260*
  estrogen and, 47
  monoclonal antibody to. See *Denosumab.*
  parathyroid hormone and, 35
  RANKL:OPG ratio, 26
RANKL inhibitor. See *Denosumab.*
Reclast. See *Zoledronic acid.*
Remodeling of bone. See *Bone remodeling.*
Renal bone disease, 271-273
Renal impairment, bisphosphonates and, 207, 273
Renal stones, calcium intake and, 162
Resorption. See *Bone resorption.*
Rheumatic and autoimmune diseases, 61t
Rheumatoid arthritis (RA), 70t

Risedronate, 180t, 193-195. See also *Bisphosphonates.*
  absorption of, 195
  action mechanism, 193
  approved indications, 180t, 193, 195
    for men, 268
    prevention and treatment of GIOP, 276
  bone mineral density, 187-190, *188-189*
  chemical structure, *184*
  dosage, 180t, 193-194
    daily dosing, 193-194
    once-weekly and twice-monthly dosing, 194
  efficacy, 180t, 193-194
    fracture risk reduction, 180t, *192*, 193-194
    glucocorticoid-induced osteoporosis, 191, *192*, 194, 276
  formulation with calcium carbonate, 195
  side effects, 180t
Risk factors for fractures. See *Fracture risk.*
Risk factors for osteoporosis, 59, 60t-62t, 63-68
  central nervous system disorders, 61t
  eating disorders, 60t, 65-66
  endocrine disorders, 61t, 66
  ethnicity/race, 11, 59
  family history, 59
  gastrointestinal diseases, 61t, 67
  genetic factors, 60t, 63
  gynecologic risk factors, 63-65
  hematologic disorders, 61t
  hypogonadal states, 60t, 86
  lifestyle, 60t, 63
  medications, 62t, 67
  modifiable factors, 63
  non-modifiable factors, 63
  rheumatic and autoimmune diseases, 61t
Romosozumab, *263*, 264
Rosiglitazone, 62t
RUNX2, 28, *29*, 34

Salmon calcitonin. See *Calcitonin.*
Salt, high intake of, 60t
Saracatinib, *260*, 261
Sarcopenia, 72
Scapular stabilization, 140

13

Sclerostin, 31, 262-264, *263*
  antibody against (romosozumab), *263*, 264
Scoliosis, 73
Screening for osteoporosis, 106-110. See also *DXA*.
  age at, 107-108, 107t
  indications for DXA, 107t, 109t
  recommendations for, 107-108, 107t, 109t
  screening tests, 106-107
Secondary osteoporosis, 43, 86-88, 267. See also *Special populations*.
  causes of, 86-88, 267
  evaluating, 87t
Sedentary lifestyle, 46-47, 49, 60t
Selective estrogen receptor modulators (SERMs), 181t, 210-214, 281. See also *Raloxifene; Tibolone*.
  toremifene, 285-286
Selective serotonin reuptake inhibitors (SSRIs), 62t, 274
SERMs. See *Selective estrogen receptor modulators*.
Sex hormones. See *Androgens; Estrogen*.
SGLT2 inhibitors, 286-287
Sialoprotein, 23
Skeleton, 19, *20*. See also *Bone entries*.
  axial vs appendicular, 19, *20*
  development in children, 269
  functions of, 19
  percentage of calcium in, 149
Smoking, 60t, 63, 70t, 280
Societal burden of osteoporosis, 11-17
Sodium glucose co-transporter-2 (SGLT2) inhibitors, 286-287
SOTI trial, 229, 230
Special populations, osteoporosis in, 267-292
  children, 268-270
  chronic kidney disease (CKD), 271-273
  diabetics, 270
  drugs that increase fracture risk, 273-287. See also *Medications*.
  men, 267-268
  renal bone disease, 271-273
Spinal fracture. See *Vertebral fractures*.
Spine. See also *Vertebrae; Vertebral entries*.
  BMD (DXA) measurement of, 90, 91-96, *92-93*

Spine *(continued)*
  compression fractures, 146
  exercise program and, 139
Src-kinase, 261
  inhibitor (saracatinib), *260*, 261
SSRIs (selective serotonin reuptake inhibitors), 62t, 274
STAR study (tamoxifen and raloxifene), 211
Steroids. See *Androgens; Estrogen; Glucocorticoids.*
Strength of bone. See *Bone strength.*
Strontium ranelate, 181t, 229-231
  action mechanisms, 229
  dosage and administration, 181t, 231
  efficacy, 181t, 229-230, 245
  indications for, 181t, 229
    as second-line treatment, 182
  long-term therapy, 245-246
  not approved by FDA (U.S.), 182, 229
  side effects and safety issues, 181t, 230-231, 245-246
  SOTI trial, 229, 230
  TROPOS trial, 229-230
Study of Osteoporotic fractures (SOF), 108
Surgical interventions
  challenges of for, 146
  indications for, 146
  vertebral stabilization, 142-146, *144*, *145*
Syncope, 68
Systemic lupus erythematosus, 269

T-scores, 81-83, 82t, 88-89
  hip, *95*
  lumbar spine, *93*
  normal, 82t, 83
  not for use with premenopausal women, 83
  reference values, 83, 89
  wrist, *97*
Tai Chi, 140
Tamoxifen, 62t, 281
  STAR study (tamoxifen and raloxifene), 211
Tartrate-resistant acid phosphatase (TRACP5b), 128t, *130*, 131
TBS score, 115, *122*

13

Teriparatide (rhPTH[1-34]), 181t, 234, 235-237. See also
    Parathyroid hormone (PTH).
  approved indications, 234, 235
    for glucocorticoid-induced osteoporosis, 276, 280
    for men, 268
    as second-line treatment, 182
  black box warning, 235, 237
  contraindications and warnings, 237, 269-270
  cost of, 182, 246
  dosage, 181t, 237
  efficacy, 235
    bone mineral density, 235, 236t
    fracture risk reduction, 235, *236*, 236t
  as recombinant human PTH, 234, 235
  side effects, 235-237
Testosterone. See also *Androgens*.
Testosterone deficiency, 44, 48
Thiazolidinediones, 62t, 270, 280
Thyroid hormones, 36. See also *Parathyroid hormone*.
  bone remodeling and, 36
  hyperthyroidism, 36, 66
  osteoporosis/fracture risk and, 62t
Thyroid stimulating hormone (TSH), 86, 87t
Tibolone, 179, 212-214. See also *Raloxifene*.
  action mechanism, 212
  dosage, 214
  efficacy, 213
  not FDA approved in U.S., 213
  side effects, 214
Tiludronate, 203
Topiramate, 67
Toremifene, 285-286
Trabecular bone
  anatomy of, 22
  changes with age, *25*
  connectivity, PTH and, 244, *245*, 246
  loss of, 43-44, *45*
  percentage in different bones, *20*, 22
  trabecular bone score, 115, *122*
Transplant anti-rejection mediations, 280-281
Treatment of osteoporosis. See *Prevention and treatment*.

Trochanter, *20*
  bone composition of, *20*, 22
TROPOS trial, 229-230
Tumor necrosis factor (TNF), 26, *28*, 48
Turner's syndrome, 60t, 66
Tyrosine src-kinase, 261
  inhibitor (saracatinib), *260*, 261

Ultrasound, quantitative bone (QUS), 106-107, 110-112, *111*
US Preventive Services Task Force (USPSTF)
  recommendation on calcium, 160
  screening recommendation, 107-108
UV-B irradiation, vitamin D and, 163, *164*

Vertebrae. See also *Lumbar spine; Spine; Vertebral entries.*
  bone composition of, *20*, 22
  deformation patterns, 114-115, *120-121*
  vertebral stabilization, 142-146, *144*, *145*
Vertebral deformation patterns, 114-115, *120-121*
Vertebral Fracture risk, prevalent fractures and, 11
Vertebral fractures, *20*, 84, 146
  asymptomatic, 11
  compression fractures, 146
  disability from, 11
  impact of, 137
  mortality associated with, 11
  pain from, 137
  pain relief techniques
    kyphoplasty, 143-146, *145*
    vertebroplasty, 142-143, *144*
  previous fractures and future fracture risk, 84, *85*
  recurrence of, 11
  vertebral deformation patterns, 114-115, *120-121*
  vertebral fracture assessment (VFA), 95, 114-115,
    116-117, *120-121*
    indications for, 114, 118t
Vertebral stabilization, 142-146
  complications of, 143-146
  kyphoplasty, 143-146, *145*
  pain relief, 143
  vertebroplasty, 142-146, *144*

13

Vertebroplasty, 142-143, *144*
  complications of, 143-146
Vertigo, 51, 68
Visual impairment, falls and fractures and, 68
Vitamin A (retinol), excess, 60t
Vitamin D, 162-169. See also *Calcium.*
  action mechanisms, 162, *164-165*
  active form ($1\alpha,25(OH)_2D)_3$, 26, *28*, 35, 162
  anticonvulsants and, 67
  assessment, 168
  biological pathways, 162, *164-165*
  bone metabolism and, 163
  calcium absorption and, 156
  deficiency, 46-47
    fall risk and, 51
    as risk factor for osteoporosis, 46-47, 60t, 63
  dietary intake recommendations, 150t-151t
  Dietary Reference Intakes for, 150t-151t
  dietary sources, 163, 166t-167t
  fall/fracture risk and, 51, 168-169, *170*
  food label, *157*, 163
  fracture reduction and, 168-169, *170*
  intake
    in children, 269
    dietary sources, 163, 166t-167t
    fracture reduction with, 158-160, *159*
    necessary for efficacy of anti-osteoporosis medications, 15
    optimal daily, 168
    recommended daily, 150t-151t, 163
      in special populations, 269, 270, 280, 285, 286
  malabsorption of, 67
  measurement of, 86
  muscle, effects on, 169, *172-173*
  parathyroid hormone and, 47
  sources and function, 163, *164-165*
  supplementation, 63, 168
    excessive, 271
  toxicity, 169

Walking, 138, 140
  back pain and, 140
  speed, fall direction and, *52-53*

Weight, 72
  low/loss, as risk factor, 62t
WHI. See *Women's Health Initiative (WHI)*.
White women. See *Caucasian women.*
Wnt ligands, 28-31, *30*
  Wnt/β-catenin signaling pathway, 28, *30*, 34, 37, 262, *263*
    inhibitors of, 262-264, *263*
      DKK1 (dickkopf-1), 31, 262, *263*
      sclerostin, 262-264, *263*
Women's Health Initiative (WHI), 182, 231
Women's Health Trial, 161
World Health Organization (WHO), definition of
  osteoporosis, 81-83, 82t
Wrist fractures, *20*, 86

Z-scores, 83, 88-89
  ethnicity database for, 83, 89
  hip, *95*
  lumbar spine, *93*
  reference values, 83, 89
  wrist, *97*
Zoledronic acid, 180t, 199-203, 285. See also
  Bisphosphonates.
  for androgen deprivation therapy, 285
  approved indications, 180t, 199, 202
    for glucocorticoid-induced osteoporosis, 276
    for men, 268
  cautions and contraindications, 203
  chemical structure, *184*
  dosage and administration, 180t, 202-203
    intravenous, 199, 202-203
  drug "holiday," 245
  efficacy, 180t, 199-203
    bone mineral density, 202, 285
    fracture risk reduction, 180t, 199-202, *200*, 201t
  HORIZON trials, 199-202, *200*, 201t
  side effects, 180t, 207, 209

13